Insights into Health and Well Being

Joe Arrigo

Number 1 Greatest Health Tip

*Watch something that makes
you laugh before going to bed.*

Preface

Following some simple health concepts will go far in achieving glowing health. Basic information about, and practicing it, is the key to preventative health care, making our visits to the doctor's office few.

This book attempts to impart critical information and dispel misinformation about health, so we may take control to make informed decisions about maintaining our most precious possession—health, rendering yourself proactive and empowered. It's the difference between preventative and curative health care. Prevention is mostly our job through our behavior and knowledge, and curative is usually our doctor's job. As a team, glowing health is within reach and available to most of us. The information herein was gathered and compiled through extensive research.

Eric Lander, leader of the Human Genome Project, denounces genetic determination, and enlightens us with the following statement, "People will think that because genes play a role in something, they determine everything. We see, again and again, people saying, 'It's all genetic. I can't do anything about it.' That's nonsense. To say that something has a genetic component does not mean it's unchangeable."

I sincerely hope you will find in these pages, information that will lead you to gaining control over, and maintaining excellent health.

Table of Contents

Cholesterol Essential for Great Health, and is Not the Mythical Boogeyman

The Hypothesis

Let us say that an inspector witnessed many large fires and noticed that at every fire, firemen were present, and therefore concluded that just on the weight of their presence, firemen were the cause of fires. This specious logic seems to be the thinking of the mainstream medical community when it arrives at the conclusion that the mere presence of cholesterol in arteries as plaque is the cause of heart disease, stroke and arteriolosclerosis—this has been the prevailing wisdom.

The American Heart Association's website states, "High cholesterol is one of the major controllable risk factors for coronary heart disease, heart attack and stroke." And, "High blood cholesterol: As blood cholesterol rises, so does risk of coronary heart disease." This is called the *lipid hypothesis*, where the only accepted therapy for heart disease was prescribing medications to lower cholesterol and severely restrict the ingestion of saturated fat, and any deviation from this

1

protocol for several decades now, has been considered heresy.

Doubts Abound

Apparently humans have consumed large amounts of saturated fats for centuries in the form of meat eggs and full-fat diary without the incidence of heart disease...up until about the 1900's. As we reduced these foods in our diets replacing them with loads of sugar, vegetable oils and processed foods, heart disease made its debut with a vengeance and became the number one killer in America. Large companies are not nefarious entities, yet it would be prudent to be cognizant of the fact that pharmaceutical and processed-food companies bring in mega-dollars as long as this hypothesis is alive and kicking; reminding me of what Sydney J. Harris wrote "There is no way of proving your point to someone whose income or position depends upon believing the contrary."

Here are some interesting facts:

- Cholesterol levels in Great Britain are the 15th lowest among 45 countries in Europe, yet they still have one of the highest rates of heart attacks

- 75% of heart attack victims have normal cholesterol

- Countries with higher than average cholesterol levels than America like the Swiss, French and Spanish have less heart disease.

Role of Cholesterol

I was quite surprised to learn recently that cholesterol is crucial to glowing health. Wow, who would ever think that, with the way we've been conditioned for decades to think otherwise.

First of all, cholesterol is an essential component in our cell membranes, and acts as an anti-oxidant where every cell in our body has the ability to manufacture it, manufacturing more or less of it based on how much of it we consume. These are some of the functions of cholesterol contributing to health:

- Enzymes convert it into vitamin D, bile salts for digesting and absorbing fats.

- Enzymes convert it into steroidal hormones like testosterone, estrogen and progesterone.

- One quarter of all cholesterol in the body is in the brain essential for synaptic health.

The membranes surrounding cells and its structure are mostly made of cholesterol helping to maintain cell integrity and communication. One-fifth of the myelin sheath coating every nerve cell and fiber is made of cholesterol. It contributes to your immune system's ablilty to inactivate more than 90% of the worst and most toxic bacterial products.

New Hypothesis

Cholesterol performs thousands of bodily functions, a crucial component for life, and many in the medical community have become aware it has suffered a bad rap as the cause of heart disease and stroke. A few years ago it was discovered that the real cause of these diseases is something called *inflammation* in the artery wall. What causes arterial inflammation? It is your body's natural defense to a foreign invader such as a bacteria, toxin or virus, and, that cholesterol being the good-guy, comes to the rescue as the fireman to put out the fire by forming a scab known as plaque over the area of inflammation.

Dr. Malcom Kendrick, author of *The Great Cholesterol Scam*, says, "Essentially cholesterol is there to help repair damage." Cholesterol is present, but it's not the perpetrator. Dr. Kendrick also saw that the MONICA study ongoing now for forty-years, shows no association with high cholesterol and heart disease.

Dr. Uffe Ravnskov, author of *The Cholesterol Myths*, goes through study after study destroying the myth that high cholesterol levels are the cause of heart disease. And, a Canadian study followed 5,000 healthy middle-aged men for twelve-years, and found high cholesterol did not at all contribute to heart disease. Another study from the University Hospital in Toronto looking at cholesterol levels in 120 men that previously had heart attacks, found that just as many men having second heart attacks had low cholesterol levels as those that had high.

This new prevailing wisdom seems to be saying in no uncertain terms, that if inflammation isn't present in the arterial walls, cholesterol levels are irrelevant, and that eating saturated fats like steak, eggs and diary bear no threat to health...and the science that says it does is very weak. Now that it's known cholesterol is not the cause of heart disease, the concern with saturated fat is, as one doctor put it, "even more absurd today."

Statins

Annual sales of statins is about $32 billion. As reported in Forbes magazine, Lipitor's lifetime sales reached $131 billion. In 2004 the National Cholesterol Education Program expanded guidelines by recommending that people who don't suffer from heart disease should take statins to prevent heart disease, increasing the number of people taking them from 13 million to 40 million. Eight of the nine people on the panel had financial ties to the drug industry.

Without side effects from these drugs, it may be justifiable to take the risk, but they're known to cause muscle damage, sexual dysfunction, and liver and nerve damage among other problems in 10 to 15% of those patients. If no inflammation is present, despite your cholesterol count being high, taking statins has zero benefit—statins should only be used for inflammation reduction, and the test to monitor inflammation is called C-reactive protein.

The Main Culprits of Inflammation

Dr. Stephen Sinatra is a convert from a pro-statin, anti-cholesterol, paid consultant of statin drug manufacturers to being a cholesterol skeptic, and is the author of, *The Great Cholesterol Myth*. He says,

> I was doing angiograms on people with [cholesterol levels of] 150 who had far advanced heart disease, and the converse, I was doing angiograms on somebody with cholesterol of 280 and they had no heart disease.

The main culprit he identifies is small dense LDL particles, making your typical total LDL number count meaningless. This is the only lipid you need be concerned about, and there is a test for it known as the *particle test*.

Another culprit is sugar, especially high fructose corn syrup. Inflammation is caused when extra sugar molecules attach to some proteins that in turn injure the blood vessel wall, and repeated injury to the wall sets off inflammation. Heart surgeon Dr. Dwight Lundell who has performed over 5,000 open heart surgeries and has looked into at least as many arteries, now is a vehement convert to inflammation being the cause of heart disease. He states,

> In twenty-five years of performing heart surgery, there was one condition that was always present in each and every patient I ever treated—that was inflammation..

and,

> When you spike your blood sugar several times a day, every day, it is exactly like taking sandpaper to the inside of your delicate blood vessels.

A third main culprit is omega-6 oils. While they are essential and part of every cell membrane, they must be in balance with omega-3 oils. Dr. Lundell goes on to say,

> If the balance shifts by consuming excessive omega-6, the cell membrane produces chemicals called cytokines that directly cause inflammation. Today's mainstream American diet has produced an extreme imbalance of these two fats. The ratio of imbalance ranges from 15:1 to as high as 30:1 in favor of omega-6. That's a tremendous amount of cytokines causing inflammation. In today's food environment, a 3:1 ratio would be optimal and healthy.

Some of the foods containing high amounts of omega-6 are corn oil, canola oil, soy oil, hydrogenated fats, margarine and shortening. One infamous example that holds a ton of this fat is French fries, of which we consume about 28 pounds each year per capita. Foods loaded with sugars and omega-6 oils for long shelf-life have been the mainstay of our diet for six decades, and are slowly poisoning us. The lipid hypothesis led to the no-fat, low-fat recommendations that created the foods now causing an epidemic of inflammation

Genesis and History of a Myth:
A Nation Embraces Junk Science

So, what was the source of this mythology? In two

words—Ancel Keys. Keys was a pathologist and diet researcher, and in the 1950s looked at the diets of approximately 13,000 middle-aged men from seven countries including the United States and Japan, where high fat intake correlated with more heart disease. In fact what he did was cherry-pick those countries which conformed to his hypothesis, and ignored all the others where data was available, 22 countries in all, where no correlation could be found. For instance, France, Italy, Norway, Sweden, Ireland and Switzerland have a high fat diet with a very low incidence of coronary disease, whereas the countries of Moldavia, Georgia, Belarus, Ukraine, Kazakhstan and Azerbaijan have low-fat intakes with a high incidence of heart disease. He used selective facts to support his theory...the worst kind of "science."

In 1957 the American Heart Association announced that a correlation between fat consumption and heart disease didn't stand up to critical examination, yet three years later altered its position despite an absence of evidence because Ancel Keys and an ally were on the AHA committee. The new report put Keys on the cover of Time magazine. Then, entrenching the "bad-fat" indictment further into the American culture, then Senator George McGovern led a committee that created a report advising Americans to eat less fat to ward off the risk of heart disease.

Even the surgeon general, C. Everett Koop succumbed to the insidious myth asserting that dietary fat was just as deadly as smoking. The U.S.D.A followed suit in 1980 issuing guidelines against fat consumption. Following that, the National Academy of Sciences reported there wasn't any valid evidence to proclaim eating less fat was more healthful. The report was promptly and soundly denounced by Capitol Hill. Then the National Institutes of Health jumped on the bandwagon saying there was no doubt that fat was the culprit of heart disease.

Ancel Keys' "research," under the guise of science, led to unhealthful dietary information and no doubt harmed many people, duping not only the people, but also the vast majority of doctors for over fifty-years now, and still persists. It's a theory that's big Pharma's best friend, perpetrating the biggest medical scam ever, with the biggest profits ever, from a class of drugs—statins.

The modern word for this virus-like spreading of presumptions is a "meme"—an automatic acceptance of supposed verified data without question.

Conclusion

While all of this may seem confusing at first, we need remember only a few things. As Dr. Lundell writes,

> Without inflammation being present in the body, there is no way that cholesterol would accumulate in the wall of the blood vessel and cause heart disease and strokes. Without inflammation, cholesterol would move freely throughout the body as nature intended. It is inflammation that causes cholesterol to become trapped.

Inflammation is the bad guy. Stay away from sugar and omega-6. And, the two tests to help us monitor inflammation are *C-reactive protein* and the *particle test.* This new hypothesis recommends using statins only as a mechanism to alleviate inflammation, not just to lower cholesterol levels—used specifically for the purpose of interfering with cholesterol levels may be detrimental to health. Also, statins aren't the only game in town to mitigate inflammation, diet modification and other life style changes such as exercise are effective as well.

A Fantasy Pill Come True: One to Replace Exercise... Oh Yea

From time to time I kid around with the personal trainers at the gym I attend asking, "When are you guys going to come up with a pill so I can stop coming here." Well folks, it's here, called SR9009.

The chemical was developed by Professor Thomas Burris and his team at The Scripps Research Institute (TSRI), one of the world's largest, private, non-profit organizations, a world leader in biomedical breakthroughs for improved health. It researches many **diseases** like cancer, Alzheimer's disease, diabetes, **obesity**, mental illness, Parkinson's disease and cystic fibrosis.

This drug significantly increased the level of metabolic activity in mice that were not allowed to **exercise**, becoming leaner, developing larger muscles, and able to run longer distances by 50%. Professor Burris explains,

> We do have indications that the effects of the drug are very similar to what you see with

someone who has metabolic disorder who starts exercising. They see a decrease in cholesterol, a decrease in triglycerides, an improvement in glucose metabolism, and a lot of this is due to transforming the muscle into a more metabolically active muscle.

SR9009 binds to a protein called Reverba, revving up metabolism and increasing skeletal **muscle** strength. Skeletal muscle is one of three types of muscle that is voluntarily controlled and are attached to bones by tendons. The other two types are smooth muscle and cardiac. "It transforms muscle into muscle that by many attributes appears to be exercising," says Burris.
SR9009 is not an appetite suppressant, laxative, fat blocker, or an ingredient found in exercise supplements, it directly works by increasing the metabolic rate and size of muscle, causing food and excess fat to be used as energy. Reverba affects muscle cells by creating new mitochondria and disposing of mitochondria that are defective, which are power generating structures within our cells that convert oxygen and nutrients into an energy chemical called ATP (andenosene triphosphate). In short, SR9009 is an exercise program in a pill.

Human Use

The results are so promising that Professor Burris and his team are pursing a biotechnology company to develop SR9009 for safe use in humans, and hope to start human trials in the next year. This poses a viable potential in answering the obesity epidemic our society now faces, requiring a lifestyle change that so few of us have been able to achieve for one reason or another. Many of the "miracle" weight loss pills now offered over the counter are unregulated and may be dangerous.

The way in which it works however, is a problem. It speeds up your biological clock. The Reverba protein targets the hypothalamus, and plays with your circadian rhythm—the master scheduler of your brain—your sleep schedule, response to light and dark, and cell production would be disrupted if you were to take the substance regularly. For short term use it would have great benefits as therapy for stopping muscle loss for bed ridden people or those hospitalized for long periods of time. Other people that can benefit enormously from SR9009 are those with severe arthritis, congestive heart failure, and COPD, where for them, exercise is not an option.

If it comes to pass that a ST9010 drug were developed, which I think will happen, making it safe to take regularly, the benefit of this drug would be for the masses; a to-good-to-be-true way of maintaining a healthy lifestyle—exercise, a swallow away. But, there is a caveat. There's no doubt many would abuse this breakthrough, using it as a free-pass to shove into our mouths greater amount of junk food and all the yummy sweets our hearts desire. There could be a counter productive blowback in response to that kind of behavior, not knowing what deleterious health effects it may bring.

I also see an irresistible attraction to this drug for those of us who do work-out and for athletes, where it no doubt would be used to enhance one's results and performance. For now, exercise is the closest thing we have to the Fountain of Youth. It is remarkably effective and transforming; well worth the investment.

A New Perspective on Cancer

New research is showing that cancer doesn't mean a death sentence. Many cancers grow so slowly they never spread to other parts of the body, some even regress naturally. As a result many current cancer screening tests are being looked at with a dubious eye. For example the U.S. Preventative Services Task Force doesn't recommend men taking the prostate PSA test saying,

> Prostate cancer is a serious health problem that affects thousands of men and their families. But before getting a PSA test, all men deserve to know what the science tells us about PSA screening: there is a very small potential benefit and significant potential harms. We encourage clinicians to consider this evidence and not screen their patients with a PSA test unless the individual being screened understands what is known about PSA screening and makes the personal decision that even a small possibility of benefit outweighs the known risk of harms.

and,

> A better test and better treatment options are needed. Until these are available, the USPSTF

has recommended against screening for prostate cancer.

Studies suggest that too many cancers don't require action—22 to 54 percent of breast cancers discovered via mammograms, and 22 to 42 percent of prostate cancers determined through the PSA test did not threaten life. Cancer researcher H. Gilbert Welch at the Geisel School of Medicine at Dartmouth says,

> The glands of the breast, the prostate, and the thyroid can all harbor a lot of small cancers that are detectable at autopsy but were not the cause of death.

The problem is it's very difficult to distinguish between dormant or aggressive cancers in their early stages, and as a result, many more treatments of radiation, chemotherapy or surgery are performed unnecessarily—an extremely serious matter, where men can lose sexual function and women their breasts, along with the psychological suffering attendant with it. What is needed are tests that can identify aggressive cancers, and research is going on in that regard. Welch says that the aggressive cancers usually manifest with symptoms rather than tests. And that, we've overstated the need to act quickly and underplayed the diagnostic value of time.

Doctors at the University of Pennsylvania have discovered the presence of a protein called Vav2 in breast tissue that may predict a cancerous condition called ductal carcinoma (DCIS) that can develop into aggressive breast cancer. Right now, two-thirds of DCIS conditions never progress into invasive cancer. Dr. Clifford Hudis, president of the American Society of Clinical Oncology said,

> which means when we treat DCIS, we are treating many people who would never have developed invasive cancer.

Improved Future Testing

Dr. Ronald DePinho at the Dana-Farber Cancer Institute in Massachusetts, is a researcher working with a new test that may determine aggressive prostate cancer better than any other testing available today. Funded by the Prostate Cancer Foundation, he and his team examined 405 tumor specimens from prostate patients, and looked for a four-gene signature. It seems these four genes excite cancer cells' ability to grow and invade other tissues. This test combined with other current tests, improved the accuracy to determine aggressive cancers to 91 percent from 84 percent.

Another promising indicator is the discovery that dormant or aggressive breast and prostate cancers can potentially be determined with biomarkers that are found in the blood or tissues of people with these cancers. The potential of these biomarkers is promising, but Dr. Hudis said it's not useful yet because it hasn't been clinically validated.

Researchers at John Hopkins are working with chromosomes. Particularly the genetic sequences at the end of chromosomes called telomeres. Telomeres protect chromosomes, and function in a way that's similar to the plastic binders at the end of shoelaces, which keeps them from unraveling. They've found that those men with short telomeres in their immune cell chromosomes are at twice the risk to develop aggressive prostate cancer. Elizabeth Platz, researcher in the department of epidemiology at John Hopkins Bloomberg School of Public Health expressed,

> We don't yet know why having short telomeres in blood leukocytes [white blood cells] seems to be associated with risk of aggressive prostate cancer. It may tell us about a person's exposure to factors that increase their risk of prostate cancer, or it may be an indication of an inherent inability to maintain telomere length, which could put them at increased risk for this disease. If so, it might be that measuring telomere length in blood leukocytes could even predict risk of many different forms of cancer.

Although these are promising protocols, at this point they are just that...promising. But given the accelerated growth of medical technology, and all technology for that matter, they're most likely closer than the horizon.

Being Less Judgmental is Being Happier

I Like You Only if You are This or That

Being judgmental is being in conflict. Conflict is not conducive to **happiness.** While judgment is necessary to guide and protect ourselves through life, using it to form opinions of people with frightening speed based on limited information doesn't serve us well.

Clarity increases when we avoid the urge of being judgmental as it helps us greatly to see what is really happening, unclouded by an indulgent knee-jerk **emotional** response. It helps us to accept those people who are not as we wish them to be, bypassing the negative wasted energy of laboring under the assumption of how people should behave and think. When we indulge in this activity, we are really becoming upset that the world is not living up to our expectations, and not a path to being happier.

We don't have to personalize the behavior of other people when it doesn't affect us. Their actions may be repulsive, distasteful or unacceptable to our standard of decorum, but just because it is, doesn't mean it's synonymous with they being wrong or immoral. Resisting this urge moves us closer to **kindness,** and kindness is an infinitely superior path to happiness. It also makes us happier because people sense our nature as easily as smelling burnt toast, and respond to us accordingly.

Being overly judgmental is the work of our ego, attempting to elevate itself above the person or group being judged as better, smarter, or morally superior; then to sanctimoniously condemn. It only satisfies the tyranny of the ego, and is detrimental to our happiness.

Separateness

In his book, *Handbook to Higher Consciousness.* Ken Keys writes these select passages.

> What do I want to change in the outside world instead of doing the inner work of changing my own response to it?

> Your ego and your rational mind labor under the harsh programming that there is a certain special way the world should be and the people around you should act—and it is up to your rational mind to put it all aright

> Whether you enjoy your life continuously, or constantly harass yourself, depends upon how well you learn to simply change what is changeable without throwing people out of your heart.

From our primitive ancestors who feared all out-
siders as a survival mechanism, tribalism seems
to be written into our DNA. We strongly identify
with the group to which we belong, and many
times suspect, even fear, others outside of it.
There are many avenues in which it can insidi-
ously seep in—racial groups, income strata, reli-
gious belief, sexual orientation, national origin,
other neighborhood, other country, etc., all of it
spelling separation from others, away from acceptance, which again, does not serve us well.

Many of us live by a set of institutional
dogmas that are hard and fast—a binary system of
good and bad—contributing to narrow thinking
with zero understanding, laying a prime foundation for harsh judgment to flourish. Taking a
closer look at those doctrines to determine if they
tend to separate you from, rather than embrace
people, will go a long way. It may be necessary to
rise above such a staunch, restrictive and biased
position.

What to Do

Since judgment comes so naturally and easily to
us, breaking the habit is difficult. Being more
aware when the urge presents itself, and perhaps
reminding yourself of some of the thoughts this
article expresses will hopefully have an impact on
changing. It will also be of great help to keep in
mind that when you are less judgmental of others,
you will also be less judgmental of yourself, increasing your self-esteem.

Know that the vast majority of people are
doing the best they can in the heat of living and
coping with life, which will tend to bring some

compassion into the game and derail the judgment impulse. We all judge, at the same time, we all love to be treated kindly. Kindness or condemnation is the choice.

If you want the truth to stand clear before you, never be for or against. The struggle between "for" and "against" is the mind's worst disease.
—Sent-ts'an, 700 A.D.

Bypassing Bypass Heart Surgery: Growing New Blood Vessels

Clogged or atrophying blood vessels starve the heart of oxygen, making the heart extremely vulnerable to heart attack, the usual treatment of which is open-heart surgery—a very dangerous procedure.

In the hope of preventing leg amputations as a result of **diabetes,** Dr. Briitta Hardy and research partner Professor Alexander Battler of Tel Aviv University's Sackler School of Medicine have developed a protein, that when injected into muscle, initiates the regrowth of tiny blood vessels which they found merge together with the rest of the circulatory system. The study funded by the Colon family here in the U.S., began by Dr. Hardy studying peptides in the laboratory; compounds consisting of two or more amino acids linked in a chain. After confirming her initial results, she then tested the synthesized peptides in diabetic

mice whose legs were dying from lack of circulation. Diabetes decreases blood circulation and
often leads to amputation of limbs. The therapy
though, rapidly reversed the constricted circulation in these mice. Dr. Hardy states,

> Within an short time we saw the formation of
> capillaries and tiny blood vessels. After three
> weeks, they had grown and merged together with
> the rest of the circulatory system.

With this procedure she completely restored the
blood vessels and saved their legs. From there the
implication was obvious—the next step was to apply it to cardiac disease, to provide new hope for
people with coronary artery disease. The results of
the study show great promise of eliminating the
need for coronary bypass surgery if blood vessels
feeding the heart can be regrown, abating all the
risks associated with it. The injectable protein
would also be invaluable for those patients suffering from the pain of angina due to blocked
arteries that cannot be bypassed or opened via
stents and angioplasty. Dr. Hardy further states,

> The biotechnology behind our human-based
> protein therapy is very complicated, but the goal
> is simple and the solution is straightforward. We
> intend to inject our drug locally to heal any oxy-
> gen-starved tissue. So far in animal models, we've
> seen no side effects and no inflammation follow-
> ing our injection of the drug into the legs. The
> growth of new blood vessels happens within a few
> weeks, showing improved blood circulation.

So, this therapy could be commercially available
soon because unlike most studies, results for
blood vessels clinically, are quick. Dr. Hardy says,

It's pretty obvious if there is regrowth or not. Our technology promises to regrow blood vessels like a net, and a heart that grows more blood vessels becomes stronger. It's now imaginable that in the distant future, peptide injections may be able to replace bypass surgeries.

This protein can also be used to protect patients with stents, acting as a coating to prevent them from developing new clots, potentially causing a heart attack. With the increased risk of stents forming blood clots, risky and expensive blood thinners need to prescribed to patients, as Dr. Hardy relates,

We could coat a stent with our peptide, attracting endothelial stem cells to form a film on the surface of the stent. These endothelial cells on the stent would eliminate the need for taking the blood thinners that prevent blood clots from forming.

Because of the nature of short time-frame of blood vessel results, we may see a revolutionary new noninvasive treatment for coronary heart disease and the elimination of amputations due to diabetic symptoms very soon.

In **America** 230,000 people undergo coronary bypass surgery each year at a cost of between $80,000 and $250,000 each, or a median cost of $165,000. That's over a $41 billion industry annually. Human nature being what it is, it's not overly cynical to suspect that we may see some resistance to this new therapy.

Doing Happiness

Scientists increasingly believe we can sculpt our brain circuitry, reshape our outlook, by understanding the reasons our brain works the way it does. Despite the programming our brains received through a millennia of trying to survive from being lunch for a host of predators, we seemingly can overcome that default setting that doesn't serve us very well in the modern world.

Two small parts of our brain structure, the hippocampus and the amygdala, helped to keep our ancient ancestors alive by alerting them of the dangers that surrounded their everyday lives. Those two glands are a part of the limbic system—the reptilian brain—that works mostly on a subconscious level to pull together bits of information, forming memories that is key to recognizing life threatening danger. The amygdala can register a "threat level red" before the conscious mind gets the message.

Because it evolved over a time when danger was rampant everywhere, we have developed a "negativity bias," alive and well with us today. Evolution favored those who were able to react with lightening speed, and we have inherited that instinct.; seemingly written into our DNA. As Dr. Rick Hanson, neuropsychologist and author of, *Just One Thing: Developing a Buddha Brain One Simple Practice at a Time,* puts it, "The brain is like Velcro for everything negative and Teflon for the positives." In his book, he presents 52 favorite simple mind actions to strengthen your neural networks toward a happier mental state.

So, burdened with this battle-hardened programmed negativity from our ancient past, how can we infuse a more lighter joyful existence? The same way you build your body by working out, the brain has the same capacity to be trained in the direction you want it to go—fundamentally it's a numbers game. We need a net surplus of cheer...that simple. The ratio is 3 to 1. Three joyful experiences to every downer. "Three to one is the tipping point that leads to a happier life," says Dr. Barbara Fredrickson, director of the Positive Emotions Lab at the University of North Carolina. It's a tipping point where you can become more resilient to adversity, bounce back from setbacks and connect better to others.

We are talking about "genuine heartfelt positive emotions," not the Pollyannaish insincere facade of "being positive," always pumping sunshine. The kind of mental states that Dr. Fredrickson speaks of are things like openness, appreciative and curious, from which spring positive emotions. In describing openness for instance, she makes us aware that all too often we're preoccupied with the past, the future, or both; rendering ourselves oblivious to the goodness that surrounds us *in the moment*—an awareness that can bring joy, dampening the insidious amygdala effect. Dr. Rick Hanson adds,

> By striving to seek out more upbeat encounters every day and savoring them to the max, you can gradually weave positive experiences into the fabric of your brain.

In addition, there is also the "facial feedback response," where simply smiling more conditions the brain away from negativity. Another powerful activity is exercise, where evidence shows that it grows neurons that are less reactive to stress. "Exercise may buffer the brain from stressful situations," says Dr John Ratey, an associate Clinical Professor of Psychiatry at Harvard Medical School and author of, *Spark: The Revolutionary New Science of Exercise and the Brain.* He advisie us,

> Think of exercise as medicine," and that, "Exercise is the single most powerful tool you have to optimize your brain function.

So, we have the tools to control and remold the "negative bias" handed down to us by our beleaguered ancestors.

No diet will remove all the fat from your body because the brain is entirely fat. Without a brain you might look good, but all you could do is run for public office.
—George Bernard Shaw

Grow Your Brain—Literally

It demands 20% of the body's blood supply and oxygen, and consumes two thirds of all its glucose. Yet it comprises only 2.5% of the body's weight. It has about 100 billion neurons (cells) and 10 trillion synapses, and the number of possible connections between them are greater than the number of atoms in the universe. The estimated total length of the branches between neurons is several hundred thousand miles, and it can store more information than all the libraries of the world. A stupendous creation, it has evolved for about 300 million years. The human brain—the only organ with the wondrous distinction of striving to understand itself, is so awesomely complex some scientists feel we will never really understand the concept by which it processes, stores, and retrieves information. It is truly a marvel of the universe.

It has been discovered the brain can actually be enhanced and grown, contrary to earlier conventional thinking, that the physical <u>brain</u> was finite. This means that not only can we alter the brain physically, but amazingly, add to its net substance. We can acquire therefore, more brain! And there are two ways in which it can be done.

The first comes from an intriguing study at the University of Illinois in Champaign by Dr. William Greenough, professor of psychology and cell structural biology. The study involved two groups of rats, each doing a distinct form of exercise. "The contrast in that particular experiment," explains Dr. Greenough, "was between animals that [had] physical exercise and animals that learned motor skills, and there were two very different effects in the two groups relative to couch potato animals. So the animals that had physical exercise increased blood vessels in the cerebellum, and we now know this is true in the motor cortex as well. The animals that exercised increased the vascular perfusion of the cortex, that is, they had more of the cerebellum taken up by blood vessels. So, that's the effect of exercise, without learning a lot of skill, as a rat by the time we test them already know how to run.

The contrast group then, had to traverse a series of elevated barriers—an elevated obstacle course—so that it took considerable skill in terms of learning to balance, learning to put their feet very very carefully in particular places, not other places and so forth. In that case the animals formed new connections in the cerebellum, new synapses (communication points) between nerve cells." He adds, "In the case of the learning, when the animals add synapses, it turns out they actually add additional components of the interconnections between nerve cells, and they add an additional amount of a supporting tissue that's called *glia.* Because of that, *the volume of the brain increases substantially."* The implications of this study seem to be profound, and when asked what those implications mean for people, Dr, Greenough states,

> I would expect the effects of skill training and exercise to be directionally similar in the human brain. Because humans have already acquired skills, there is going to be a lot of circuitry that's already been altered in the brain, nonetheless I would expect exercise to have effects on brain vasculature if it was maintained for some period of time, and I would expect motor skill training to have effects on brain synaptic formation and circuitry.

There are many exercises that involve both aerobic and motor skill training such as jumping rope, tennis, racquetball, fencing, boxing, etc. The raw endurance of these activities will generate new capillary proliferation in the brain, carrying more blood, and with it more oxygen and glucose as fuel for better performance. The process of acquiring the skill inherent to the activity creates new circuitry along with the supporting tissue (glia), necessary to accommodate it. Another option is to participate in two distinct forms of exercise separately, for instance running for vascular formation and tai chi for motor skill training; or fast walking combined with learning the tango. As to how long it takes for these new formations to occur within the brain, Dr. Greenough points out, " The regimen in the original study was four weeks, but we now know that at least some molecular changes are taking place very very rapidly."

The second way to increase brain circuitry is to pursue intellectual challenges. This encompasses a very broad spectrum, whatever tickles your fancy. Opening yourself up to new concepts, new philosophies, crafts, new games such as bridge or chess, another language, music, becoming computer literate, and on and on. In a published research paper written by Dr. Greenough and Dr. Craig Baily at the Center for Neurobiology and Behavior, Columbia University in New York, they cite a study in which a fixed sample of the occipital cortex from rats living in a cage filled with toys providing mental stimulation, weighed more than a group placed in standard cages or reared individually. The augmented tissue volume was due to increased interconnections and synapses.

The implications of this revolutionary research portrays the brain as eagerly awaiting our input so it may organize and amplify its structure. The brain is indeed a marvelous machine, and now, even more so in light of its ability to adapt and recreate itself. The thought that by building our bodies we are literally building our brains brings a new meaning to physical activity, and is a quintessential illustration of the mind-body connection, in that physical health and mental health are far more inextricable than we ever imagined.

Muscling In on Youth: Aging Biomarkers

Ten Biomarkers of Aging

The two most important aging biomarkers are:

Muscle Mass and Strength

The remaining eight are:

•Body fat   •Metabolic rate   •Blood sugar tolerance • Bone density   •Aerobic capacity •Blood pressure   •Cholesterol /HDL ratio •Body temperature regulation

The good news is they are all within our control. Muscle mass seems to be the Holy Grail of youthfulness since it directly controls most of the other markers—strength, body fat, metabolic rate, blood sugar tolerance and bone density.

We just need to know that muscle is the furnace for calorie consumption called your metabolic rate at rest, which in turn has a direct effect on the amount of body fat you carry—fat is metabolically inactive. Muscles also make your body more efficient at burning sugar, lessening the burden on your pancreas to manufacture insulin in order to counteract excess sugar in the blood.

Actually, all it takes is a couple times a week at the gym totaling about an hour to an hour-and-a-half per week. Muscles are very responsive; they'll gladly give you back whatever you invest into them

We lose 6.6 lbs. of muscle each decade after young adulthood. The body tends to lose half its muscle and double its fat by age 65. Two scientists at Tufts University, William Evans and Brian Rosenberg, wrote the book, *Biomarkers,* and found that these declining markers, through weight resistance training, can be reversed even in older people. They in fact maintain that building muscle is the key to rejuvenation for the elderly.

The most efficient way to use weights in resistant training is to use enough weight where you can only do about 5 to 6 repetitions. Research shows this increases metabolism by another 8% than by doing more repetitions with lighter weights. As a bonus, as I've experienced, within four months your strength will increase by an astounding 50% over and above a standard program of 10 to 12 repetitions with lighter weights.

The second most important biomarker? Strength; a natural by-product of weight-training, as is bone density since they are stressed as the muscles pull on them during resistance training. So, to recap; building muscle mass increases strength, metabolic rate, and bone density; decreases body fat, and makes the body more efficient at burning off excess sugar. A little aerobics improves the remaining four.

Evans and Rosenberg also tell us that muscle mass and strength rejuvenates the entire physiology and overall vitality, definitely slowing down the aging process. They write,

> Heredity isn't everything, after all. It's certainly possible for a well-maintained Volkswagen bug to last longer than an abused Mercedes.

Longevity Genes

There what is known as longevity genes called sirtuins.. There are seven of them, and they have a significant effect on the rate of our aging process by regulating almost all cellular functions. Activating these genes helps to reverse metabolic decline, enhancing a longer healthier life.

Exercise has been found to activate and enhance at least one of the sirtuins, promoting the production of new healthy mitochondria, which in turn, boosts energy production.

NAD:
Most Important Molecule in the Body

Nicotinamide adenine dinucleotide (NAD) is one of the most if not *the* most important molecule in the body, as it is required for over 500 chemical reactions to regulate almost all major biological processes.

The human body is made up of at least 37 trillion cells, and they all contain and rely on NAD to perform their functions. Every one of them needs NAD. Without this molecule we would die.

NAD turns nutrients into energy. So it's essential to the creation of energy we receive, and is a key player in metabolism. As part of the aging process, our supply of NAD declines.

So, what does this have to do with exercise? As it turns out, exercise stimulates the production of NAD in our bodies. Dr. David Sinclair is a biologist who is a professor of genetics and co-director of the Paul F. Glenn Center for Biology of Aging Research at Harvard Medical School, and his book *Lifespan: Why We Age and Why We Don't Have To,* is on the New York Times best sellers list at the time of writing this book, The Sinclair research group is a world leader in the understanding of why we age and how to reverse it. His research shows that exercise increases the production of NAD, and affects DNA repair. This is very exciting news that shows exercise actually has a profound impact on retaining our youth.

Conclusion

The Scottish physician of the 18th century Dr. William Buchnar said,

> Of all the causes which conspire to render the life of man short and miserable, none have greater influence than the want of proper exercise.

I fully acknowledge it's difficult to start and especially sustain an exercise program, it's a drag. Do it anyway. I do, because the benefits are enormous. A small investment into exercise reaps big returns. It would be like buying Amazon stock at $5 a share. Muscle up.

Poor Sleep, Obesity, and Diabetes

Today, more than 30% of men and women between the ages of 30 and 64 have reported sleeping less than six hours per night. In 1960, a survey conducted by the American Cancer Society said Americans slept about eight hours a night, but in 1995 a National Sleep Foundation poll showed that number had dropped to seven hours. Interestingly, the dramatic uptick of obesity and diabetes in the U.S. has occurred over the same time period that sleep duration has declined. In fact, obesity and diabetes are increasing at an alarming rate worldwide, particularly in the U.S., and many researchers are looking at sleep deprivation as one of the major players in the phenomenon.

Researh has shown there are three main pathways where not sleeping long enough for long periods of time can cause these diseases.

- *Alterations in Glucose Metabolism*: Keeping the narrow range of our blood sugar in balance in avoiding both hypoglycemia and hyperglycemia is crucial to staying alive, and sleep has been recognized for almost 15 years as playing an important role in glucose regulation. Losing sleep destabilizes the regulation of glucose, and if sleep loss becomes chronic, it increases the risk of developing diabetes

- *Appetite Regulation:* The regulation of appetite is controlled by two hormones, *leptin*, which is appetite inhibiting; and *gherlin*, which stimulates appetite. In a laboratory study, men were subjected to only four hours of sleep for six nights which decreased their mean leptin levels by 19%, and increased their gherlin levels by 28%, therefore increasing their hunger and appetite.

- *Decrease in Energy Expenditure*: Energy expenditure, of course, plays a major role in body weight, and people with sleep deprivation report a substantial reduction in energy and physical activity. And there is good evidence that leptin seems to increase energy expenditure, while gherlin decreases it.

As you can see there is a combination of factors at work here in concert against our best interests, perhaps producing a synergistic effect in increasing the chances of developing obesity and diabetes. The diagram below is a visual representation of the process.

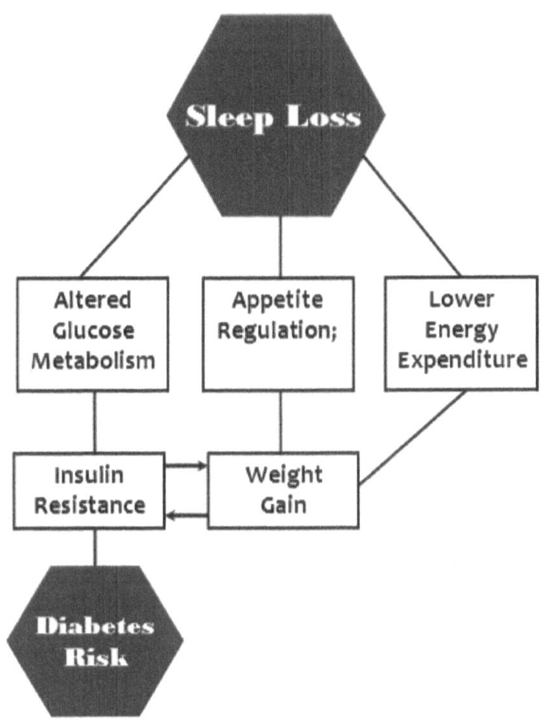

Studies in Spain, Japan and the U.S. have shown a pronounced association between shortened sleep duration and being obese, where data collected from the American Cancer Society indicated weight loss occurred when sleep duration was increased, as did the Wisconsin Sleep Cohort Study in 1995, and the Nurses Health Study of over 80,000 women.

Dr. Eve Van Cauter

Dr. Eve Van Cauter from the University of Chicago, and a specialist in the effect of circadian rhythms (a daily biological activity influenced by the environment like the alternation of day and night) of the endocrine system, was the first to discover that sleep deprivation impacts appetite and secretion of insulin, leptin and ghrelin, inducing insulin resistance which causes higher risks of obesity and diabetes. She has conducted numerous studies where short-term sleep restriction lowered the levels of leptin, the hormone that signals the body it's had enough to eat, promoting larger intakes of food.

Although researchers say many more studies need to be done, it seems the handwriting is on the wall that getting more sleep can have a major impact on curbing the epidemic of obesity and diabetes. The Wisconsin Cohort Study showed that a about seven-and-a-half hours of sleep per night was most effective in bringing down BMI (Body Mass Index).

Conclusion

It seems that chronic sleep loss has become the new norm for scores of people due to our fast paced society, and perhaps all that's needed is behavior modification to get back on track. A lot of good things take place during sleep—the body renews tissues, forms new blood cells, and releases growth hormone, and the brain undergoes a myriad of renewal functions.

Sleep is an active and dynamic state that impacts our waking hours to a great extent,

and its process of rejuvenating us must be given
the proper amount of time so we can be our opti-
mum selves both physically and mentally.

Take a Breather: Regenerate with Good News

The amygdala. An almond shaped mass located deep within the brain, is in large part responsible for the survival of our distant ancestors. It's fire-alarm function is a warning system alerting them of impending danger, like potentially being an appetizer for some stealthy predator, or of the scary others from another tribe that might pose a threat. Those alarmist type impulses emanating from the amygdala are still alive and well within all of us today, and we need to be aware that it is a biased little bugger. It embraces bad news, and treats good news as an afterthought. As Dr. Rick Hanson, neuropsychologist and author of, *Just One Thing: Developing a Buddha Brain One Simple Practice at a Time,* puts it,

> The brain is like Velcro for everything negative and Teflon for the positives.

The amygdala served *Homo sapiens* well in primitive times, but can become a liability in the modern world as it affects our thinking, what we emphasize in our lives, and at worst, define our attitude about existence. So, let's give this group of neurons in our brain a healthy dose of well needed therapy, step back, and look at the big picture for some good news.

Longevity

We are living longer. But it gets better—we're also living healthier, even the elderly. David Cutler, the Otto Eckstein Professor of Applied Economics at Harvard University and author of a study based on the Medicare Current Beneficiary Survey said,

> Effectively, the period of time in which we're in poor health is being compressed until just before the end of life. So where we used to see people who are very, very sick for the final six or seven years of their life, that's now less common. People are living to older ages and we are adding healthy years, not debilitating ones.

A recent Danish study also showed that today's older people are more alert and cognitive than previous generations. Most likely, the heightened awareness of healthy foods, exercise and maintaining active brains are contributing to this trend.

Crime

In 2014, the FBI released statistics compiled from the first six months of 2013, reflecting a decrease in reported violent crimes and property crimes in America. It said murders are down 6.9 percent, rapes down 10.6 percent, assaults decreased 6.6

percent and robbery down 1.8 percent from 2012. And author of *The Better Angels of Our Nature: Why Violence Had Declined*, Harvard social scientist Steven Pinker says,

> Violent deaths of all kinds have declined, from around 500 per 100,000 people per year in prestate societies [tribal rather than governmental} to around 50 in the Middle Ages, to around six to eight today worldwide, and fewer than one in most of Europe.

In the United States between 1993 and 2012, homicide, robbery, assault and rape dropped by an astounding 48 percent. Even more amazing, New York's violent crime in that same period, dropped by 71 percent. What are some of the reasons that may be causing this? Probably the most obvious reason is there are far more prisoners than ever before. It's estimated that about one-fourth of the overall decrease is impacted by incarceration. The law enforcement technique of hot-spot policing is another, where the great majority of crime seems to emanate from the same venues, and specifically placing police in those areas utilizing computerized maps has been very effective in reducing crime.

Surprisingly, another reason for the decline in the crime rate is medical. People whose blood has been contaminated with lead tend to be more aggressive and violent. Protection from the Environmental Protection Agency came in 1974, when regulation prohibited big oil from adding lead to gasoline, and simultaneously, lead in paint was also banned. Lead in Americans' blood then fell by four-fifths between 1975 and 1991, and economist Jessica Wolpaw Reyes maintained that the absence of leaded gas led to violent crime being cut in half during the 1990s.

Poverty

The really good news here is the 2013 Human Development Report that tracks the progress of countries using the Human Development Index (HDI), scoring countries by its standard of living, education and healthcare. It reports that between 1990 and 2008, the percentage of impoverished people declined by half, from 43.1 percent to 22.4 percent. It's an historic drop in the poverty rate. The report states,

> Never in history have the living conditions and prospects of so many people changed so dramatically and so fast.

All the rated countries have improved their HDI score since 2000. The greatest gains came from China, Brazil and India. with excellent progress in countries like Uganda, Bangladesh, Ghana, Rwanda, Tunisia, Vietnam and Laos. In the past three decades the number of people that live on less than $1.25 a day, decreased dramatically from half the developing world to 21 percent. In the last fifty years the world has grown far better than the previous five-hundred. The following is a synopsis of some of the great things that are happening in our world.

- Global income has tripled in the last 50 years.

- There's been a 30 percent increase per capita in food supply.

- We're at the lowest time of homicide ever since the Middle Ages.

- Literacy rates across the world have increased from 25 percent to 80 percent.

- Infant mortality rates around the world have declined by 99 percent.

- In the same period, human life span has doubled.

- The number of major wars declined from 37 in the mid 1980s, to about 26 today. And Steven Pinker writes, "Today we may be living in the most peaceable era in our species' existence.

- For the first time in history, slavery isn't legal anywhere on the planet.

Keep in mind as you read, watch and listen to some of the horrors of the daily news, that your amygdala is basking in it, favoring it, nudging your mind to be weighted in that direction.

Are GE Foods
Harmful Frakenfoods?

Some refer to them as Frakenfoods. They feel it is a sin against nature, a dangerous mutation that will cause the consumer physical harm, and should be labeled as a GE food. Genetically engineered plants are created in the laboratory where they have changes introduced into their DNA altering their genetic makeup and then tested for the desired qualities. Directly tampering with the DNA of food unnerves many people, yet over a trillion GE meals have been served without a single illness.

Detractors' attitude rests on the belief that agriculture is natural, but in fact, *all* crops are genetically modified; mutations that are designed to yield unnaturally large yields, so says Matt Ridley, biologist and author. The orange color in carrots is due to a mutant first discovered around the 16th century in Holland. The banana is a seedless sterile mutant, and now struggling to fight off pests and diseases, lacking the genes to fight back, and could be doomed. And wheat descended from three wild grasses, unable to survive as a wild plant...there is no wild wheat. GE has given us a quantum leap in the information we have, and really allows us to understand exactly what we're doing.

A good example of how GE foods are beneficial is the Hawaiian papaya industry which was facing a collapse because of the deadly papaya ringspot virus. Genetically modifying it made it resistant to the virus and was a savior to the industry, and now 80% of Hawaiian papaya is genetically engineered.

Here are some of the great advantages of genetically engineered foods:

- GE appears good for the environment. The seeds don't require plowing, so the soil structure remains in tact, halts erosion, and improves carbon sequestration.

- Substantially increases yields.

- Dramatically decreases the use of pesticides, herbicides, fossil fuels, and nitrogen laden fertilizers helping to save our ravaged oceans from further severe damage by the runoff of these chemicals. Runoff has turned our coastal waters into dead zones so severe that the U.S. must now import 80

percent of its seafood from abroad. Nitro-
gen-rich fertilizers and waste, strips ocean
areas of oxygen, causing what is known as
hypoxic dead zones. There are now more
than 500 zones.

- Will soon have crops that can grow in
  drought and saline environments.

- Crops can be fortified with protein, vita-
  mins, minerals, made to be virus resistant,
  lower natural cyanide content, and longer
  storable times; improving the health of
  millions of people.

- Frost tolerance. An antifreeze gene from
  cold water fish has been introduced into
  plants such as tobacco and potato. With
  this antifreeze gene, these plants are able
  to tolerate cold temperatures that normally
  would kill unmodified seedlings.

In 1996 there were 1.7 million hectares of biotech
crops; by 2010 it increased to 148 million hectares, making it the fastest crop technology in the
history of modern agriculture. (Hectare = 10,000
square meters. Equivalent to just under 2.5
acres).

Taking a Second Look at GE Foods

When I wrote the previous chapter, *Are GE Foods Harmful Frakenfoods?*, my daughter Andrea messaged me saying, "Hi Dad, Just read your article...It would be cool as a follow-up to this article to write about the disadvantages of GE as you just wrote about its benefits," along with an attached academic article (my children keep me honest). So, along with that attachment, I did some further digging to arrive at the following.

First of all, here is a list of some common GE foods:

Corn
Soy

Sugar
Aspartame
Papayas   GE papayas have been grown in Hawaii since 1999, and can't be sold to countries in the European Union.
Canola   One of the most chemically altered foods in the U.S.
Cotton
Dairy
Zucchini
Yellow Squash
Tomatoes

More than thirty other foods are now being tested in field trials such as apples, bell peppers and coffee. The Environmental Working Group analyzed data from the U.S. Department of Agriculture finding that each American consumes about 193 lbs. of GE foods annually, and the average American adult weighs 179 lbs., eating more than their average weight each year. That breaks down to 68 lbs. of beet sugar, 58 lbs. of corn syrup, 38 lbs. of soybean oil and 29 lbs. of corn based products. Children and Hispanics are most likely eating more than that since they eat more corn based products from corn flour. The first GE food was introduced in 1994, the tomato, so the long-term effects of humans consuming these foods remain unknown. That is a paramount point—we don't know—and seems to be going full steam ahead, but there is some preliminary evidence as we shall see.

The reason this research isn't being conducted independently is because under the law, those companies that hold the patents like Monsanto and Dow, get to decide in most cases what testing can and cannot be done. How cozy. Having companies test their own products for safety is like appointing Bernie Maddoff to head the SEC. They are only required to complete 90 day rat feeding trials to determine safety. These companies seem to also have great power and influence within the government, and probably in bed with the USDA. That's not much of a surprise to most Americans since our insane system allows money to move Congress. Monsanto has reported profits at $4.5 billion for 2019; that's a lot of grease to easily buy just about any legislation it wants. As Jay Leno once said, "The economy is so bad, Merck had to lay off 3 senators." One thing we *do* know—corporations have a miserable track record when it comes to choosing truth over profits.

The Details

Roundup® is a Monsanto herbicide product that's used on Roundup Ready® crops, meaning the seeds are genetically inserted with an enzyme which renders them resistant to Roundup, while surrounding weeds are killed when soy crops are spayed with it. That's very profitable for Monsanto since farmers have to buy the herbicide when they buy the seeds. The question is whether this enzyme is harmful to humans. Monsanto claims that because people cook soybeans before eating them. it deactivates the enzyme rendering it harmless, however, raw soybeans are fed to cattle, and many people eat medium rare or rare steaks making it conceivable they will ingest the functional enzyme. And, since these plants are engineered to be resistant to Roundup, it allows farmers to spray with wild abandon—its use has increased by an estimated 383 million lbs., between 1996 and 2008. Saturating the crops with this stuff helps me to sleep easier at night. So, we get a twofer—the enzyme and more of that savory herbicide.

Enter the French Study

France has completed the first long-term study of GE's led by Gilles-Eric Seralini of the University of Caen. He and his colleagues used a Monsanto seed variety known as NK603 to resist its Roundup product. The study was published in *The Food & Chemical Toxicology Journal*, titled "A Comparison of the Effects of Three GM (genetically modified) Corn Varieties on Mammalian Health." The study used 200 rats fed a lifelong diet of Roundup genetically modified corn over a period of two years, and found they developed large tumors and had severe liver and kidney damage. The first detectable tumors occurred 4-7 months into the study—50% of the males and 70% of females died prematurely, while 30% of males and 20% of females died prematurely with a conventional diet.

While I don't adhere to scare tactics, I would be remiss in not citing this study because it's the only long-term study ever done with GE foods, and Monsanto seems adverse to doing such a study. As one researcher, Dr. Michael Antoniou said, "I am shocked by the extreme negative health impacts." Russia has temporarily banned Monsanto's genetically modified corn as a result of this study linking it to cancer.

However, the French food safety authority ANSES decided not to ban the corn, stating that the study didn't support its claims linking the product to the devastating results of the rats, yet they call for more studies like it and Seralini stands by his research.

What to Do

Since this is a contentious issue and Monsanto is fighting back attempting to discredit the above study, we, rather than passively waiting to see how it all turns out, can do to a few things to protect ourselves. First and foremost substantially decrease your high fructose corn syrup intake...Americans consume far too much of it; a great deal of it coming from soda. We can also buy our produce from local markets and farmer markets rather than big chains, or if you can afford it, U.S. certified organic foods. There is no doubt that labeling by law is the most protective thing the government can do to give people a choice, something that GE manufacturers are resisting. What's the logic of that?—keep the people in the dark so they're unaware of what they're buying, means higher profits. Over 50 countries have implemented labeling GE foods including Mexico, Australia, Japan, Russia, India, South Korea, United Kingdom, Germany, China and Brazil.

The people of California voted on Proposition 37—the Mandatory Labeling of Genetically Engineered Food Initiative, that would have make them the first state to give its residents the power of choice. It failed.

Professor Richard Lewontin, Professor of Genetics at Harvard University says,

> An ecosystem, you can always intervene and change something in it, but there's no way of knowing what all the downstream effects will be or how it might affect the environment. We have such a miserably poor understanding of how the organism develops from its DNA that I would be surprised if we don't get one rude shock after another.

And, Dr. Judy Carman, Epidemiologist, of Flinders University in Australia writes,

> Independent testing of these foods is urgently required, incorporating long-term animal and human experiments. As these would take years, it would be wise to place a moratorium on these foods for 5 years...To do otherwise could be likened to permitting a giant feeding experiment on millions of people.

Since the makers of GE foods have enormous power with the government, it's more likely that Mitt Romney will have Spam and Cheetos for dinner tonight than a moratorium be put in place, therefore, labeling is the only game in town, and must be put into law for the good of the people and future generations.

The Marketing of Disease to Our Children

The Centers for Disease Control and Prevention (CDC) tells us that by 2050, 1 in 3 adults in the United States will have diabetes if current trends in children's diets continue. What's driving this oncoming train wreck? The power of the food, beverage and fast food industries and their lust for fatter bottom lines.

The food and beverage people spend about $2 billion a year marketing unhealthy foods to children, and the fast food moguls spend about the same amount directed at our kids, and 98% of the nearly 4,000 food-related ads children watch each year are for products high in sugar, fat and salt—now 40% of their diets. What could possibly go wrong?

To exacerbate that, in 2010 the food and beverage industry spent more than $40 billion lobbying (bribing) Congress to vote down regulations among which would decrease the marketing of unhealthy foods to kids. As an example of their nefarious slight-of-hand, a study in 2007 conducted by the Prevention Institute found that over half of the most aggressively marketed foods that strongly suggest having fruit in them by picturing fruit on the package, contained no fruit whatsoever.

Legislation

The Inter-agency Working Group (IWG) is an agency that includes the Federal Trade Commission (FTC), the Centers for Disease Control and Prevention (CDC), the Food and Drug Administration (FDA) and the United States Department of Agriculture (USDA). In 2009 Congress commissioned them to develop standards in advertising foods to children, where it stated that food ads directed at children must provide, "a meaningful contribution to a healthful diet," and that those foods in the ads to children must, "contain at least 50% by weight one or more of the following: fruit; vegetable; whole grain; fat-free or low-fat milk or yogurt; fish; extra lean meat or poultry; eggs; nuts and seeds; or beans."

General Mills retorted that under the IWG guidelines, most foods now purchased by consumers would be classified as unhealthy, saying, "of the 100 most commonly consumed foods and beverages in America, 88 would fail the IWG's proposed standards." That's an admission that most of what kids are eating is crap! General Mills also related that if everyone in the country ate healthy, it would cost them $503 billion a year. Well hey, we wouldn't want them to sacrifice that revenue stream over a trivial matter like children's health...how then could they pay their CEO Jeff Harmening almost $8 million a year?

It's not difficult to understand how Congress is in bed with the food and beverage industry—the industry spent $37 million buying Congress to trash the IWG recommendations.

The Big Three

The food industries' food scientists and executives from companies like PepsiCo, General Mills, and Nestle know and utilize to its full extent, that sugary, salty, fatty foods are addictive, targeting the same pleasure centers of the brain as cocaine does, and, if they hook young kids, they will be customers for life. This works. For instance, when I make potato salad, I found that adding some sugar to it along with the normal amount of salt, it's more delicious.

In his book, *Salt Sugar Fat*, investigative reporter Michael Moss asked these food scientists and executives if they drink soda or feed their children Cheetos and Lunchables (prepackaged trays of bologna, cheese and crackers); their answer—no. Howard Moskowitz, the man who reinvented Dr Pepper, told Moss, "I'm not a soda drinker, it's not good for your teeth."

Moss also writes about a 2008 Kellogg's commercial for Frosted Mini-Wheats where they claimed, "A clinical study showed kids who had a filling breakfast of Frosted Mini-Wheats cereal

improved their attentiveness by nearly 20 percent," but half the children who ate it showed zero
improvement in attentiveness. These companies
are lacing, what would be considered wholesome
foods like yogurt and spaghetti sauce with loads of
sugar and salt, such as Yoplait with twice the
amount of sugar as Lucky Charms, and a half-cup
of Prego Traditional spaghetti sauce with as
much sugar as three Oreos and one-third the daily
recommended salt intake.

In Conclusion

As long as we have a system where Congress can
be greased, we will have corporations with deep
pockets controlling the playing field, much to the
detriment of the people. The game is rigged.
Even the innocence of our children, the most vulnerable among us, are no exception to the greed
that pervades our economic and political system.
For that reason, we must be vigilant in what goes
into our children's tummies.

The Toxin that is Sugar

Americans consume about 150 lbs. of sugar annually, much of it coming from the 57 gallons of soda we each guzzle annually. One hundred years ago we consumed 10 lbs. What's it doing to us? Some pretty bad things. There is sucrose, glucose and fructose. The worst among these? Fructose, especially High Fructose Corn Syrup (HFCS), ubiquitous in almost every manufactured food like soda, fruit juices, cereals, ketchup, jellies, graham crackers, bread crumbs, etc. Look for products that don't include it like Hunts Ketchup instead of Heinz, Heio jelly instead of Smuckers or Welches, and get Trader Joe's Bread Crumbs instead of buying Progresso. Above all, stay away from soda which is loaded with it.

The first to know is that sugar causes us to eat more in three ways, as it interferes with three hormones—ghrelin, leptin and dopamine—all of which give us the feeling of hunger satisfaction, signaling to our brain that our tum-tum is busy metabolizing what we just ate and to cease putting more food in our mouths. So, by ingesting sugar, we're hungrier.

Then there is a condition known as metabolic syndrome, where the cells in your body ignore the action of insulin, otherwise known as insulin-resistant. When that occurs, the pancreas respond by manufacturing more insulin and eventually can no longer keep up with the demand leading to what diabetologists call "pancreatic exhaustion," otherwise known as diabetes. Further, chronic elevated insulin levels in the blood leads to higher triglyceride levels, higher blood pressure and lower levels of HDL cholesterol (the good stuff), and, worsening insulin resistance, or metabolic syndrome—the perfect storm for heart disease.

So, what causes metabolic syndrome? Researchers like Peter Havel and Kimber Stanhope at the University of California, are finding that it's caused by the accumulation of fat in the liver. And what causes fat in the liver? Researchers have demonstrated that by feeding animals enough fructose is an easy way to do it. Stop feeding them fructose, and the fatty liver promptly disappears, along with insulin-resistance.

Havel and Stanhope have actually done studies on humans where they've given healthy people three high fructose corn syrup sweetened cans of soda a day, and found the liver starts producing fat within two weeks, but it's important to point out that this isn't acute toxicity, it's chronic toxicity, having negative effects over a long period of time, yet the consequences are nevertheless devastating. This is really bad stuff.

Long term studies still need to be done, but given the research to date, and the unprecedented rise in obesity and diabetes, it would be prudent to get the sugar out of your diet now, especially when given the fact that every researcher has already done so. So, if high fructose is on the label, put it back on the shelf.

The Upside of Sadness

Sadness has always been associated with undesirable, something we try to overcome, get beyond, and transition into happy. While happy is the state we all would like to be in, there now seems to be upsides to being in the state of sad.

Joseph Forgas is a psychologist at the University of New South Wales, and just published the article, *Don't Worry, Be Sad! On the Cognitive, Motivational, and Interpersonal Benefits of Negative Mood*. We are not talking about debilitating lengthy bouts of severe depression, just the sad moods most of us experience from day to day living. Through his research he's discovered that negative moods do have an upside, several in fact. So, let's look at them.

- Ironically, there's a motivational aspect to a sad mood. The odds are that more sad

- people persist in doing a difficult job, where happy people are more likely to abandon a challenging task.

- There is a phenomenon in psychology called the *primacy effect*. If you were presented with several traits of another person, you would remember and be impressed most with the first trait presented to you. For instance, if you were told that Sam was intelligent, sensitive, outgoing and opinionated, you would remember him as an intelligent person; if the list were read to you in reverse order, you would remember Sam as opinionated; and, a happy mood enhances that bias, however a negative mood removes it, exhibiting that sadness enhances judgment.

- The *dictator game* is an economic psychology study where there are two players. One player receives a dollar amount, say $25, and that person can distribute it any way he or she wishes. If you propose giving the other person $5 and you keep the rest, and the other person says no, both of you receive nothing. It's an emotional negotiating scenario to determine if a deal could be struck, and the psychological interplay it manifests. It was found that sad people made more generous offers being fairer, where happy people, again ironically, were more susceptible to their demanding ego.

- Forgas believes that sad people are more accurate and perceptive in their observation of the world around them. Researchers found that sad people who witnessed an episode, held true to what they witnessed when they were subjected to a misleading line of questioning, and happy people were more vulnerable to being nudged into false memory.

Being skeptical is another trait of sad people, being less likely to be gullible in accepting myths with a more heightened awareness of insincere people.

- In a very interesting experiment, Forgas found that sad people were more resistant to stereotyping people. In a game called *shoot don't shoot*, the object was to shoot bad guys holding guns, but to refrain from shooting when the people were holding a beverage or a cell phone, where half the targets wore Muslim type turbans. All tended to shoot more at the Muslim image, but that tendency was magnified with the happy people.

These are some of the surprising and fascinating results of Forgas' research, typifying how mysterious the human psyche is. Our goal of course shouldn't be sadness for these advantages, it's simply good to know that in the normal course of life where our brain chemistry vacillates from one day to the next and life's disappointments affect our moods, you can go along with it as part of being human and abandon the notion that we always must feel happy all the time.

It also affords an opportunity to reflect and reevaluate our recent actions and if appropriate apply some beneficial changes, which wouldn't occur if we were perpetually skipping and singing wearing a permanent Cheshire smile.

Using the Placebo
Effect to Heal

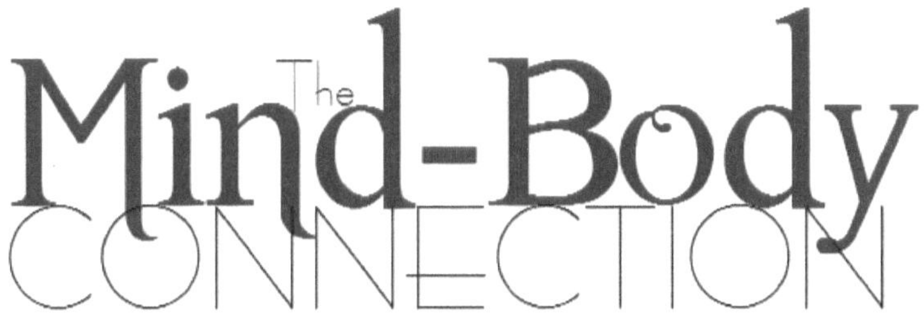

The placebo effect is a mechanism that triggers the vast power of the mind to affect the body in positive ways. It's so effective it's the main reason researchers need to employ a double blind approach in studies when testing the efficacy of drugs to deliver an intended and meaningful result, whereas the placebo effect would be the standard by which the drug is measured. The placebo effect is the irrefutable evidence of the mind-body connection.

Some Examples

In a study at Ruhr University Bochum in Bochum, Germany, more than 1,100 patients underwent treatment for back pain. One group received real acupuncture, the second was fake acupuncture where the needles were inserted randomly on the body at a shallow depth, and the third received medications or other types of Western treatment. After six months the patients were polled—the real acupuncture group enjoyed a 47 percent improvement in pain relief, the fake acupuncture group had an *impressive 44 percent* improvement rate, and the third only 27 percent.

Psychologist Irving Kirsch, Associate Director of the Program in Placebo Studies at Harvard Medical School, doing an analysis of 47 trials of six of the most widely prescribed antidepressants, discovered that 82 percent of patients given a placebo pill instead of an antidepressant, had an improvement in mood duplicating the effects of the antidepressants.

Forty-six asthma sufferers were given either an inhaler with the drug albuterol or with a saline solution. Researchers measured how much air the patients could inhale and exhale over twelve visits before and after treatment, and those that were treated with albuterol increased their respiratory scores by 20 percent, while the others using saline solution increased only 7 percent, however, when the patients were asked what their respiratory discomfort was on a scale of 0 to 10, everyone except those that didn't receive any treatment at all, reported a 50 percent improvement.

Despite the fact that the drug had a substantial physiological medical effect, patients perceived no difference between *it* and the placebo, which could mean that the placebo effect activates a mechanism that is distinct from the pathway of drugs yet equally effective. Irving Kirsh says, "A medical treatment has two components, the actual pharmacological effect and the placebo component of the active treatment."

The distinct and separate brain path of the placebo effect signature has been supported by neuroscientists using positron-emission tomography to map the brain's response to pain, and similar tests using MRI showing that additional brain regions are activated.

Incorporating the Placebo Effect into Treatment

Since the placebo response have a distinct pattern of brain activity that can be differentiated from the one medication utilizes, they offer a separate and unique therapy. The question is how can doctors utilize this untapped powerful treatment without deceiving the patient like surreptitiously prescribing placebo pills?

Well, there seems to be two ways. Ted Kaptchuk is a researcher and director of the Program in Placebo Studies with Irving Kirsch. His team did a study of 262 patients with irritable bowel syndrome (IBS), assigning them to either a placebo acupuncture (fake), or a waiting list. They also subdivided the placebo group into patients who received no conversation with the acupuncturist and those patients who received a generous amount of attention and empathy with the practitioner.

Those acupuncturists who listened intently to each patient, repeated his or her words, expressed confidence, touched the patient, and also became silent for about 20 seconds in deep thought, had a large impact on their patients. The results? Of the waiting list group, 28 percent reported their IBS symptoms improved, those receiving the fake treatment and near zero doctor-patient interaction, a 44 percent improvement, and those who received close empathetic attention, a 62 percent improvement. So, *the bedside manner **is** the placebo.*

Secondly, it's possible that fake pills and procedures could be used without deceiving the patient and still work. Kaptchuk and Kirsch with their team, did a study in 2010 where they gave 40 patients with IBS placebo pills, but the patients were informed they were placebos. They described the pills as,

> placebo pills made of an inert substance like sugar pills that have been shown in clinical studies to produce significant improvement in IBS symptoms through mind-body self-healing processes.

Taking the placebo for 21 days, these patients reported feeling better overall with less severe symptoms than the 40 patients receiving no treatment.

These techniques used with empathy, incorporates the potent placebo effect into medical practice to the great benefit of patients. Ted Kaptchuck expresses, "It is really turning the art of medicine into a science of art."

*Skepticism may prevail and hypnosis
may remain underused because of the
tendency to doubt or fear of the unknown.*
—Dr. James H. Stewart

What is the Role of Hypnosis in Medicine?

What Actually is Hypnosis

Basically, it is an induced state of mind in which our normal critical, judgmental, biased and skeptical nature is bypassed, a state of relaxed highly focused attention, allowing for the acceptance of suggestion, induced with cooperation from the patient. It may be surprising to know that it is a natural state of mind, similar to being absorbed in a book, or lost in a movie, and daydreaming.

Hypnosis is a window into which the very powerful subconscious mind is rendered receptive to suggestion, where the conscious mind is distracted and dormant, and perhaps contrary to what many people perceive about hypnosis—an alert state of mind, not at all related to sleep or unconsciousness, and is in fact a waking state. Hypnosis is not merely a process of following in-

71

structions as you would see performed on stage entertaining an audience, it is an actual change in the brain's perception exhibited by tests of people undergoing hypnosis.

For instance, volunteers were placed in a hypnotic state and evaluated using positron emission tomography (PET). When given the suggestion to see color, the color perception areas of the cerebral cortex were activated as they were looking at color or black-and-white color patterns. When given the suggestion to see black-and-white, the color perception areas of the brain showed decreased activity regardless of what the subjects were viewing, demonstrating hypnosis actually changes the brain's perception.

How it Started

Hypnosis began with the Austrian physician Franz Anto Mesmer in France in 1778. In the 19th century, English surgeon John Elliotson and Scottish surgeon James Esdaile performed hundreds of surgical procedures using only hypnosis as the anesthesia. It was the same time that both ether and chloroform became popular, displacing hypnosis as anesthesia.

Hypnosis in Medicine

We all possess the power to heal ourselves as our bodies fight off illness every day. Hypnosis is a vehicle to tap into and enhance that power residing within the subconscious, managing illnesses with less medication or none. Unlike a procedure or medication, hypnosis is not something administered to you, rather, its healing power comes from within; the hypnotherapist being only a guide to reach it.

It seems hypnosis is an underutilized therapy in medicine—in 1958 the American Medical Association published and approved a report from a two-year study by the Council on Medical Health indicating there is "definite and proper uses of hypnosis in medical and dental practice," recommending the establishment of "necessary training facilities" in the U.S. The American Psychiatric Association said, "hypnosis has definite application in the various fields of medicine," and a panel from the National Institutes of Health issued the statement that there is "strong evidence for the use of hypnosis in alleviating pain associated with cancer."

So, what are some of the potential applications hypnosis offers patients?

- **Pain......**The fact that hypnosis has been successfully used as an anesthesia for surgery for over a century speaks volumes. Clinical trials showed significant pain relief in patients with burns and jaw pain. It also relieves pain caused by chronic headache and back pain.

- **Irritable Bowel Syndrome (IBS)...**In a 1984 study in England, thirty patients with IBS were randomly selected for seven individual hypnotherapy sessions, all of which showed significant improvements with no relapses at a three-month follow-up; and very good results with hypnosis for

IBS have been confirmed in many other trials.

- **Peptic Ulcers......**Thirty patients with recurring peptic ulcer disease were randomly treated with either ranitidine or hypnosis whereby they were all healed. After twelve-months of monitoring only 53% of the hypnosis group experienced relapse compared to 100% of the ranitidine group.

- **Obstetrics......**As reported in the article *Hypnosis in Contemporary Medicine* by Dr. James H. Stewart of Mayo Clinic, "Hypnosis as anesthesia for childbirth has a long successful history supported by several trials."

- **Oncology......**The nausea and vomiting associated with chemotherapy has been lessened with hypnosis in children as compared to the control group.

- **Tinnitus (Ringing in the Ear)..**Patients with chronic tinnitus improved significantly with hypnosis.

- **Asthma......**A study of 55 asthmatic patients used bronchodilators less frequently and had less wheezing than control groups. One study showed that 21% had become symptom free and were able to discontinue medication.

- **Smoking......**In 1992 an analysis of smoking cessation involving 633 studies and

72,000 participants, hypnosis was the most successful method.

- **Impotence......**Many trials have shown impressive results for treating nonorganic impotence with hypnosis. One trial comparing hypnosis with a placebo group, showed an 80% improvement in sexual function to only 36% with the use of a placebo.

- **Dentistry......**Hypnosis relieves pain, anxiety, speeds up the perceived time of the procedure, and minimizes bleeding and gagging.

- **Obesity......**Obesity is a complex problem involving emotional behavior where hypnosis has had limited success. Several studies have shown that hypnosis enhanced the success of weight loss over other methods not using it, and also in conjunction with them. Certainly it would make sense to consider hypnosis before any type of surgery is considered.

Conclusion

One would think with all the data available regarding the efficacy of hypnosis, far more doctors would be working in conjunction with hypnotherapists as a first line of attack for many diseases in light of its noninvasive nature. It seems there still remains some stigma about hypnosis, much to the loss of the patient. As more people become aware of the potential it offers, it will empower them to explore that potential. According to Dr, Stewart, acceptance is increasing as a result of "careful, methodical, empirical work of many pioneer researchers," but he also writes, "Nonetheless, skepticism may prevail and hypnosis may remain underused because of the tendency to doubt or fear of the unknown."

Hypnosis is a testament to the mind-body connection, supporting the irrefutable fact that they both constitute one eloquent inextricable mechanism, and should be treated as such. At this moment the National Institute of Health (NIH) is funding clinical trials of complementary and alternative medicine, and hypnosis is one of its focuses. Because of this effort, hypnosis may become a greater part of mainstream medicine, and taken full advantage of by health care providers, as it affords a harmless, noninvasive and viable treatment option.

Why Do Exercise Programs Fail? Getting a Handle on Success

The vast majority of people who begin an exercise program, abort it within a very short time frame. Their good intentions and exuberance is a timid and highly ineffective match for the reality of consistent physical effort. Exercise bestows us with some wonderful and profound health benefits, but that awareness alone is not enough to sustain the discipline a long-term workout program demands. So, how do we achieve stick-to-it-tiveness? As with forming any strategy, one must look at the entire concept of an exercise program and determine what the objective is. The objective here is not just to start a program of exercise—anyone can start one—we want longevity, ongoing action; and we do it by changing our behavior from the inside out—from the psyche to the body. We base our behavior modification program on a successful, true and tried, never failed us, human trait—*laziness*. We   want   to   circumvent enthusiasm and rely upon laziness. Sound paradoxical? Perhaps. Until we see that laziness offers us an opportunity to condition ourselves without relying on frail and fickle enthusiasm which abandons us quickly like an over inflated balloon when it gets near heat and pops. This will put the odds dramatically in our favor to succeed long-term, remembering that the definition of success is to maintain, sustain, and uphold what we are starting; where the value lies in carrying on, not over-doing it for a couple of weeks or months then fizzle like a short fuse.

Ideally exercise should be a habit, where we define habit as an action we perform without conscious thought. Unfortunately, few of us attain that level of automatic action as it relates to exercise because it requires great effort exacerbated by being boring, requiring conscious thought before you can gear up for action; and the only action that that thought will induce is regurgitation. We can though, shoot for the next best thing—*psychological addiction*, which is achievable. It's a state of mind that exerts a force over our behavior that is in most cases more powerful than our natural inclination to resist exerting effort.

For instance, you come home from work, you're tired, maybe drained, your motivation is barely twitching and enthusiasm is undergoing the death rattle. You are experiencing a feeling, a powerful feeling that devastates any thought of physical exertion before it evens begins. Your feeling is saying, *"Are you kidding Flash? Let's eat and find the remote."* But then, you find yourself changing into your athletic clothes, preparing for a workout. That's psychological addiction. It's a behavior. It's a feeling of cheating and denying your best interests. Notice I'm saying *feeling*, not logical thought. Only a feeling can overcome another feeling, whereas rational thought doesn't have a prayer.

With this process there's rarely a mental war of self-motivation, rather a powerful conditioned behavior dynamically promoting action regardless of the initial feeling. It is a nemesis to laziness, using laziness to defeat laziness by following a logical path. So, how do we become psychologically addicted? Through conditioning, through long term behavior. But haw can long-term behavior be achieved if *long-term* and *exercise* is a contradiction in terms? The answer is— *easy effort*; with *short duration*. Easy and short duration is a concept to condition the mind. The process looks something like this:

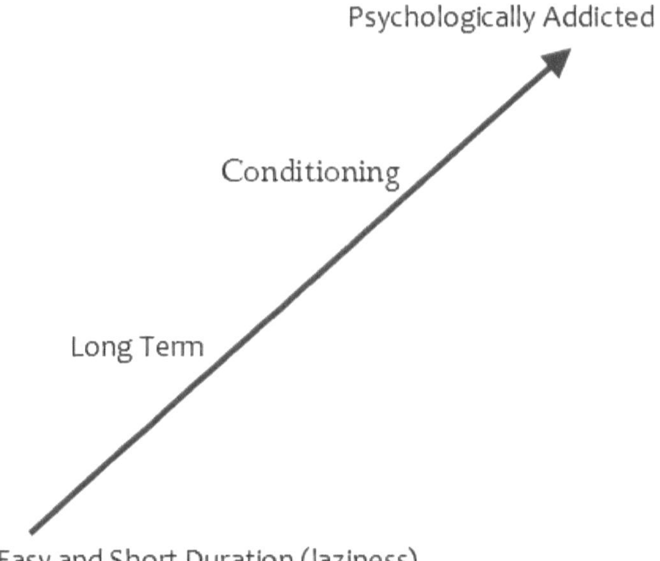

Since we can't start with psychological addiction, we need a substitute, and easy and short does it until psychological addiction starts to take hold. We'll rely 95% upon easy and short with gradual increase, and 5% on self-discipline. This is infinitely more in line with long-term success. Relying on self-discipline and enthusiasm from the very onset for a full-blown workout program is a recipe for failure, where enthusiasm will short circuit conditioning by doing too much too soon, and therein our undoing lay waiting. *Note*: Too much doesn't mean you can't handle a program physically, it means you cannot emotionally sustain it.

The mental and emotional aspect of ourselves needs to be addressed first—it is the foundation for success for a prolonged program. This is a way to keep yourself centered, and psychologically in balance as it relates to this program. Becoming excited about starting something new is great, but one must be optimistically cautious because our emotions play tricks on us. Enthusiasm puts us off-center, a position of disadvantage in terms of long-term success. It's common sense to know that a person who starts out real, knowing what it takes, has an enormous advantage over someone starting with stars in their eyes, especially when we know that the vast majority of people who engage in an exercise regimen fall by the wayside in short order.

Since we're speaking about adding something to your life that will contribute mightily to your long-term health and youthfulness, it's imperative to manipulate the odds in your favor from the start. There are a plethora of how to workout books and video tapes all showing their nifty routines. None that I know of address this most crucial aspect of dealing with long-term success. Except for the most disciplined among us, the yippy-yi-o-you-can-do-it approach doesn't work, because as it is written, "The spirit is willing, but the flesh is weak."

A detailed description of an exercise program itself is beyond the scope of this chapter, but generally you can pick five exercises such as push-ups, curls, pull-ups, squats and sit-ups. Then a cardiovascular activity like walking. Start with 3 repetitions each for the exercises, and walk for 1 minute. Do that twice a week on specific days of your choice. Do that regimen for 2 weeks, then increase the repetitions and time you walk to 2 minutes for another 2 weeks. The following chart is a suggestion of the pace to guide you. After reaching the last entry on the chart, you can begin doing 2 sets of 10 reps for each exercise, or stay at that level if you're satisfied. Once you reach that level of conditioning, you can customize the program as you wish, and be pretty confident you'll continue it.

	Exercises	Cardio
2 weeks	3 reps each	1 minute
2 weeks	5 reps	2 minutes
2 weeks	5 reps	3 minutes
3 weeks	8 reps	4 minutes
3 weeks	9 reps	5 minutes
3 weeks	10 reps	6 miuntes
3 weeks	10 reps	7 minutes
4 weeks	10 reps	10 minutes

This strategy and program is supported by a basic tenet of exercise, which says, a little effort goes a long way. The effort-to-reward-ratio is high, an offer difficult to refuse. By exerting a little effort, very little in the beginning; will dissipate any intimidation you may feel, and you'll soon feel in control.

Our society is not in very good shape, and that includes more and more of our children. In a sedentary, fast paced, fast food society where obesity and stress are epidemic, directing our energies to the priorities that can be the most effective in rejuvenating and enriching our lives is paramount—what gives the most bang for the buck. And few investments can compare with the enormous return exercise offers us.

Enjoy Nuts,
Coffee, and Alcohol:
A Case for Living Longer

We've all heard the phrase, "Everything that tastes good is bad for you." Well, here's exceptions to the rule. Serious studies have found nuts, coffee, and alcohol actually extends longevity—how great is that?—pleasure *and* health.

Nuts

The least surprising among these is nuts, as we've all heard of their healthful properties. They contain unsaturated fats, omega-3 fatty acids, fiber, vitamin E, plant sterols and L-arginine; and as reported by the Mayo Clinic, lowers low-density lipoproteins (LDL), reduces the risk of developing blood clots, and enhances the health of the lining in the arteries. The studies that have confirmed the life-prolonging effects of nuts was published in the prestigious New England Journal of Medicine. One study conducted by the Nurses'

Health Study (1980-2010) among 76,464 women, and another by the Health Professionals Follow-up Study of 42,498 men (1986-2010). During those periods, 16,200 women, and 11,229 men died, finding that those consuming nuts inversely impacted their mortality rate.

Eating nuts once per week led to a 11 percent reduction in mortality, a 13% reduction eating them twice a week, and a whopping 20% reduction in mortality eating nuts seven or more times a week. The studies showed,

> Significant inverse associations were also observed between nut consumption and deaths due to cancer, heart disease, and respiratory disease.

Since nuts are high in calories, they should be consumed in moderation—the Food and Drug Administration recommends about a handful a day (1.5 ounces).

Coffee

Coffee is one of the most heavily consumed beverages in the U.S., and its health liabilities vs. its benefits have been controversial for decades. The New England Journal of Medicine published a study conducted by the National Institute of Health—AARP Diet and Health Study of 229,119 men and 171.141 women between the ages of 50 and 71 that were not suffering from cancer, heart disease or stroke.

After adjusting for those who smoked and any other unhealthy behaviors, "There was a significant inverse association between coffee consumption and mortality." For men who drank one cup per day the reduction in mortality was 6 percent, for those who consumed 2 cups per day the mortality reduction was 10 percent, and 12 % reduction consuming 4 or 5 cups per day. For women, the respective reductions were 5 percent, 12 percent, and 16 percent.

The study's conclusion was that the consumption of coffee resulted in an overall reduction in deaths.

Alcohol

The health benefits of alcohol consumption will for most people, be a surprise, yet it's not really new knowledge, since the well known Framingham Heart Study of the 1970s found that drinkers had less incidence of heart disease with moderate alcohol consumption. But in 1974, Harvard investigator Carl Selzer was prohibited from publishing those results by the National Institute of Health, which actually funded the study. So it seems, that any news of health benefits derived from alcohol consumption is suppressed because of a strong anti-alcohol bias in the U.S. Another example happened in 2007, when PBS produced a show called *The Hidden Epidemic: Heart Disease in America,* with a panel of experts moderated by Larry King, never discussed the impact on health from moderate drinking, ignoring the subject altogether.

It must be noted here though, that with alcohol use there is a higher incidence of deaths due to injuries, violence, suicide, poisoning, cirrhosis, and some cancers, but a lower rate of death due to heart disease. Once again there was a nationwide study published in the New England Journal of Medicine, and conducted by the American Cancer Society with 251,420 women and 238,206 men participants 30 years or older, from 1982 to 1991. Of the total participants there were 46,000 deaths. The overall conclusion of this study is that the "rate of death from all causes were lowest among both men and women who reported one drink daily, the rates were about 20 percent below those of nondrinkers. Above one drink per day the overall death rate among drinkers increased," and "have concluded that moderate alcohol consumption reduces the overall risk of cardiovascular disease."

The one seemingly contradiction I found in the study was "the rate of death from breast cancer was 30 percent higher among women reporting at least one drink daily than among nondrinkers." The finding that is most astounding is *"in the subgroup that is at highest risk for cardiovascular disease (60-79 years old with preexisting risk factors), the rates of death from all causes among drinkers remained significantly below those among nondrinkers, even for subjects reporting four or more drinks daily."* So, the risk is greater for this group not to drink at all, than to drink too much.

In one other study—the Harvard Professionals Study—where the participants were doctors of normal weight, nonsmokers, exercised and had good diets. The study found, even in this healthy group, the same reduction in heart attacks of those who had one drink daily.

Conclusion

The data definitively shows the health benefits of consuming these three items, and especially with alcohol, is counterintuitive. The data is king, and should not be overridden by what we might think is socially acceptable or taboo, or cling to a belief we embrace dearly, if we are to behave in ways that are clearly in our own best interest. It would also be reasonable to expect the beneficial impact on health to be synergistic if all three were consumed on a regular basis. Moderation is key.

Making Hard Choices.
It's Not a Science

What career should I choose, should I have children, who to marry, should I live in the city or the country? Choices such as these may pose hard choices for many. What technique or perspective can we utilize to become more competent in making hard choices, and alleviate the agonizing stalemate of paralysis by analysis? Is there an element we fail to factor in that leaves us immobilized in coming to decision?

Well. it seems there is. Philosopher Ruth Chang of Oxford University has astutely drilled down to what the underlying and insidious problem is—what it is we're missing, what we're assuming. She feels that we've misunderstood hard choices and the role they play in our lives, that to understand them is to uncover a hidden power we each possess and that we're looking in the wrong place for the answers, mainly out there, rather than from within. With an easy choice, one option is clearly better than the other. With hard choices, one is better in some ways, and the other in better in other ways. One is not better than the other, they are on par—like should I uproot my life to go on to a better job, or stay here with what I'm comfortable with?

We think of hard choices as big decisions, but not necessarily so. Chan gives an example of deciding what to have for breakfast as a small choice. Should I have bran with fruit, or a chocolate donut. One is far healthier...the other tastes a hell-of-lot better. One is not better than the other overall. Realizing that we can come to decision on these smaller choices, makes the bigger ones look less intimidating and problematic, and we'll be less likely to be tempted to take the safest least riskiest options the primary factor for making that hard choice.

Because there is no *best* option, is precisely what makes them so difficult to deal with. So, the first rule when deliberating hard choices is to liberate yourself from the erroneous perception that one is better than the other overall. And as Ruth Chan points out, since they are on par, doesn't mean we now merely flip a coin...that's not a viable method for deciding something important to your life. The choices, after all, do have merit.

The conundrum arises when we make the unwitting assumption that values like kindness, justice, what gives us joy, and empathy are comparable to scientific measurement like weight and length. As Chan expresses,

> We tend to assume that scientific thinking is key to everything of importance in our world.

Values and scientific quantifying are of different worlds. Eloquently, she enlightens us that the world of *what is,* is not the same as the world of *ought.* Of the three quantifiers of worse, equal or better, we normally use to decide, cannot apply to on par choices. We now need to introduce a fourth new dimension—values—to replace worse, equal or better. This realization now empowers us to create and infuse our very own reasons into the hard choice to be made. Chan posits a scenario where we live in a world where all choices are easy choices, either better or worse, therefore it's all rational, where we would of course pick better over worse. This world of easy choices would enslave us to reasons, period, *dictated to us* by simple a-b-c logic, a binary robotic-like selection of on or off. Rather when we face hard choices, choices that are on a par, we are then afforded the opportunity to *create* reasons for our choice, not dictated from outside ourselves, but from within.

When choices are on a par, seeking information that would tell you if you're making a mistake is futile because it doesn't exist, giving you the power to create reasons for yourself guided by the human values that mean the most to you, injecting yourself into the equation of choice, recognizing and validating reasons from within you, not from out there—this is who I am— *I am the author of my life.*

Chan says there are drifters, that is, people that allow the world to write the story of their life, allowing mechanisms like reward and punishment or fear to guide the drumbeat of their lives, away from their authentic selves. In Ruth Chan's words,

> Hard choices are precious opportunities for us to celebrate what is special about the human condition. That the reasons that govern our choices is correct or incorrect sometimes run out, and it is here in the face of hard choices that we have the power to create reasons for ourselves, to become the distinctive people that we are. And that's why hard choices are not a curse, but a Godsend.

This unique concept of difficult decision making, humanizes the process and our choices, enhancing our freedom as we integrate who we are into our path in life. It is truly empowering to see them as opportunities to be true to ourselves.

Convictions are more
dangerous enemies of truth than lies.
—Friedrich Nietzsche

Belief Systems and Health

John F. Kennedy said,

> The great enemy of truth is often not the lie—deliberate, contrived, and dishonest—but the myth—persistent, persuasive, and unrealistic.

These convictions come from belief systems; something we all have in one form or another. A belief system can be thought of as the mental acceptance of a proposition, statement, or concept as true on the grounds of apparent authority, which does not have to be based on actual fact. Many of these beliefs, ideas, or convictions have been programmed into us since childhood, many of them without any basis of reason, where hope and wishful thinking are mistaken for knowledge; and become powerful because they are a large part of our identity, and thus have great influence over our lives.

Looking at health, if a person has a belief that says genetics is the only factor that dictates health, and never examines if that is really true, he or she will most likely miss the opportunity to enhance his or her health and have a more enjoyable life. If they allowed themselves to look at some hard information about vibrant health, they will discover that behavior is the primary determinant to their physical status, not genetics, they then are much more likely to take control and create a much healthier, joyful life. Leader of the Human Genome Project, Eric Lander, denounces genetic determinism with the following quote,

> People will think that because genes play a role in something, they determine everything. We see, again and again, people saying, "It's all genetic. I can't do anything about it." That's nonsense. To say that something has a genetic component does not mean it's unchangeable.

Belief systems are usually rigid rather than flexible, narrow rather than broad, closed rather than open, and immobilizing rather than liberating. When left unchecked, our strongest belief systems can blind us to reality, and become one of the great impediments to empowering ourselves and problem solving.

It is our belief systems that we use to make judgments about the world and about any given situation as being true, good, bad, happy; where we become so emotionally invested in protecting them, facts to the contrary are rendered invisible; seeing only what aligns with and supports our beliefs. They tend to make us think in binary terms, either right or wrong, good or bad, moral or immoral, whereby knee-jerk conclusions are drawn; painting things with a broad brush into gross generalizations in a frail and lazy misguided attempt to simplify the complexities and nuances of life.

The conscious mind may want to make logically precise decisions, yet the unconscious mind wants to feel good. There are times when we know down deep that we are in conflict with our own intellect and common sense when defending our beloved belief system. We turn our back on, and abandon our intellect in order to cling to, and protect, our precious ideological comfort zone, disallowing ourselves to know what we know. If we resist and dismiss that "annoying" nudge, and doggedly continue along the same path of thought out of shear pride and allegiance, we dishonor and deny our intellect, our inner voice, and the integrity of our true and better selves. Neuroscientist and brain researcher, Paul MacLean laments,

> You know what bugs me most about the brain? It's that the limbic system, this primitive brain that can neither read nor write, provides us with the feeling of what is real, true, and important.

The operative word in Dr. MacLean's quote is *feeling,* infused with certainty based on our belief, then becoming our option to either engage our intellect as to the veracity of that feeling, or just blindly and passively ride with it. Intransigent belief constructs a mental barrier to further knowledge and understanding; where nothing, not even irrefutable evidence, will cause it to consider or yield to that information. A great example of this in action happened when I was watching the Rachel Maddow Show airing from Alaska in

2010 when Joe Miller was running for Senator. She interviewed some of his supporters on the street protesting against Eric Holder the Attorney General, regarding and opposing his position on gun control as they perceived it. She asked one woman holding up a Joe Miller campaign sign,

> "Can I just ask, why are you upset about Eric Holder?"
> She replies, "I know that he is anti-gun."
> Rachel, "What has he done that's anti-gun?"
> The woman then utters these vacuous words, "I *don't have all the facts* but I *know* that he is anti-gun."

Rachel asked a man participating in the rally the same question; he replied,

> "I don't know enough about that to answer that truthfully, Rachel."

These people who behave solely from the feeling they receive from their limbic system that Dr. Paul MacLean depicts in the above quote, do so without the slightest inclination of pausing or questioning it with their intellect, and gather information. This immediate functionality of the limbic system served our primitive ancestors well ensuring their survival by allowing them to react swiftly in the face of imminent death, bypassing the slower conscious assessment of a perilous situation, providing an instantaneous interpretation to environmental stimuli—no conscious thought necessary. This primitive responsiveness lives within us still, and doesn't serve us well interpreting modern world problems unless we make the effort to consciously assess those feelings bubbling-up from our primitive brain.

Bertrand Russell, one of the twentieth century's most influential intellects, insightfully recognized the unchallenged power of the limbic system when he wrote,

> [I]t is curious how people dislike the abandonment of brutish impulse for reason.

And, Mark Twain observes,

> The trouble with the world is not that people know too little, but that they know so many things that ain't so.

It takes courage to be uncertain because doubt leaves the door open, and openness to investigation leaves us vulnerable to the unknown, where the renunciation of absolute certainty is the most difficult step toward intellectual freedom. The 18th century French philosopher Voltaire said,

> Doubt is not a pleasant condition, but *certainty* is an absurd one.

As enlightening and insidious as Dr. MacLean's insight is, we nevertheless have the ability to identify our own illogical fallacies, and can therefore, if we choose, manage them with deliberation—we can disown flawed beliefs and replace them. And yes, it requires considerable fortitude to challenge long held beliefs; they are comfortable, perhaps loyal to a particular group, familiar, and cherished, and can even conjure up warm memories of the way it was, carrying the baton for the people we love or loved. Beliefs can also come from self-serving bias, self-deception, and fuzzy thinking; in short, an integral part of the culture in which we were raised and conditioned. When we dare to challenge them we feel the fear of the unknown as we venture beyond what we previously established as our safe boundaries. We must take heart, however, and remember that the realm of the unknown is precisely the place where solutions to unsolved problems are found.

As Ayn Rand points out in her book, *Philosophy: Who Needs It,* we all need a philosophy,

> Your choice is whether you define your philosophy by a conscious, rational, disciplined process of thought—or let your subconscious accumulate a junk heap of unwarranted conclusions [and] false generalizations...

There are huge dividends in examining our beliefs and putting forth deliberate effort of sound, reflective thought—it brings us closer to the truth—though it can be frightening. This does not mean we abandon our intuition...our inner voice; it does mean we use it along with *good information,* and in doing so; we open up the potential to become both more competent and more liberated. Acting on knowledge works far better than acting on belief. Alexander Green writes,

> Genuine faith is belief in the absence of evidence, not belief in spite of the evidence.

Another example of belief is one that is told to children; that if they don't receive good grades they won't be successful in life. If that child, after internalizing this limiting belief, in fact *does* finish school with poor grades, he or she is much more likely to accept that success is something they cannot achieve...a self-fulfilling prophecy; when in fact, many eminently successful people didn't get good grades in school, and many multi-millionaires never finished school. Some notables are Walt Disney, Bill Gates, Mary Kay Ash, Mark Zuckerberg, Woody Allen, Steve Jobs, Michael Dell, George Eastman, Benjamin Franklin, Quentin Tarantino, Richard Pryor, Peter Jennings, Henry Ford, Richard Branson, and John Rockefeller Sr. Then there is geneticist and entrepreneur, John Craig Venter, who has developed the first artificial self-replicating cell in the lab—artificial life, and one of the first who mapped the human genome; carried Cs and Ds on his eighth-grade report cards, and says he was a horrible student in high school, not good at any subject material. It wasn't until he became a medic in the Navy serving in Vietnam that he was inspired to return to school and pursue a career in medical research. He was named in *Time* magazine's list of the 100 most influential people in the world in 2007 and 2008. Human beings are far more dynamic, profound, and complex to have their potential, worth, and spirit measured solely on the basis of school grades.

In his book, *What Intelligence Tests Miss*, Keith Stanovich describes the mental temperament that leads to highly effective cognitive effectiveness,

> The tendency to collect information before making up one's mind, the tendency to seek various points of view before coming to a conclusion, the disposition to think extensively about a

problem before responding, the tendency to calibrate the degree of strength of one's opinions to the degree of evidence available, the tendency to explicitly weight pluses and minuses of a situation before making a decision, and the tendency to seek nuance and avoid absolutism.

Removing and replacing these restrictive, even enslaving beliefs with good information would have a massive positive impact on many peoples' lives. Hard and fast belief systems tend to make us react automatically to certain new information...sort of a robotic reflex-action, similar to the fight-or-flight syndrome, circumventing our invaluable intellect to analyze objectively; where new information bypasses the intellect, surrendering it over to the primitive brain, similar to a short circuit in an electrical system which bypasses the functional circuitry. That mechanism, left unchecked, locks us into a mental state, surreptitiously slipping by our awareness that we *do* have a choice. And choice is our greatest power.

Developing the fortitude to hold those beliefs up to scrutiny removes the sentry at the gate of our minds whose role it is to filter out all information that doesn't align with, protect, and caress our old beliefs. I remember watching supermodel and actress Lauren Hutton in an interview on the *Johnny Carson Show*, when she stated that she's attracted to men who exhibit *mental bravery,* that is, men who are unafraid to admit when they're wrong, or will intrepidly hold their beliefs up to scrutiny and reassess their position when they are presented with compelling information. Their intellectual honesty was appealing to her because she perceived them as secure and strong enough as men to face down their male egos and welcome thoughts differing from their own that exhibit merit.

Belief systems edit our reality and can be a barrier to discovery, especially when they mutate into an ideology or dogma, causing us to distrust any idea that is outside of its doctrine; limiting us from learning. In conceding to dogma, we close off our most precious gift—our minds—to new evidence, forfeiting our choice to be a free thinker. Dogma being the petri-dish which cultivates un-thinking, where your views are arrived at by default, denying yourself the liberty of forming and asking critical questions endeavoring to mine for truth; to unveil an untruth.

We wholly empower ourselves by becoming free thinkers. It's of paramount importance that we are prepared to detach from our belief systems when we recognize good information screams foul, because they govern our behavior and de-termine our decisions through life; being on constant vigil for what we *want* to believe is true, isn't the driving force for *what* we believe is true; and entails pausing, and consulting our intellect, always. The bottom line is developing the courage and authenticity to be *intellectually honest with ourselves.*

Life is such an enigma with all its para-doxes, ironies, and convoluted twists, when at times even common sense becomes counterintui-tive to truth. With infinitely more unknowns than knowns, none of us is privy to what life really is, and because of that, none of us comes remotely close to possessing ultimate wisdom to always know the truth, therefore, it is imperative that we each continually reevaluate our belief systems in order to protect our thinking from becoming ossified; keeping in mind that veracity not only involves accepting as true or not accepting as true, but also in suspending judgment.

What you believe, and why you should believe it, is in actuality a scientific question; believe because it is supported by evidence and verified by experiment, believe it because years of substantiation has given it credence...believe it because your *intellect* tells you it's true, while being prepared to modify your position if new evidence arises.

With all the contentious issues before us such as health care reform, global warming, and abortion, a safe bet we can all count on is that the truth lies somewhere between the two conflicting views. And perhaps "believe" is an inappropriate word to use, rather "just follow the evidence" serves us far better.

Bertrand Russell enlightens us with these profound and provocative words about the courage of honest thought,

> Men fear thought as they fear nothing else on Earth—more than ruin, more even than death. Thought is subversive and revolutionary, destructive and terrible, thought is merciless to privilege, established institutions, and comfortable habits; thought is anarchic and lawless, indifferent to authority, careless of the well-tried wisdom of the ages. Thought looks into the pit of hell and is not afraid...Thought is great and swift and free, the light of the world, and the chief glory of man. But if thought is to become the possession of many, not the privilege of the few, we must have done with fear. It is fear that holds

men back—fear lest their cherished beliefs should prove delusions, fear lest the institutions by which they live should prove harmful, fear lest they themselves should prove less worthy of respect than they have supposed themselves to be.

Our health is dependent upon acting in accordance with good information, not our treasured beliefs. We all need to honor and revel in truth, and rely on the gift of our intellect and the courage to use it in leading us there, "The greatest obstacle to discovery," says historian Daniel Boorstin, "is not ignorance—*it is the illusion of knowledge.*"

Guns as a Health Issue, and,
The Three Psychologies
of Guns

Gun violence is a leading cause of premature death in the U.S., killing more than 38,000 people and causing nearly 85,000 injuries each year. Gun violence is complex and deeply rooted in our culture. The Small Arms Survey stated that U.S. civilians alone account for 393 million (about 46 percent) of the worldwide total of civilian held firearms. This amounts to 120.5 firearms for every 100 residents.

The Centers for Disease Control (CDC) is our nation's top agency to research public health issues. Yet, for years, stemming from the Dickey Amendment, the one area that has not received funding and attention is gun violence. The Dickey Amendment, passed in 1996, mandates that "*none of the funds made available for injury prevention and control at (CDC) may be used to advocate or promote gun control.*" The amendment was introduced after the National Rifle Association lobbied Congress in response to a CDC-funded 1993 study that reported that guns in the home were associated with increased risk of homicide in the home. Is gun violence a public health issue? Many Americans would have different answers to this. The truth is, it's a complicated issue that brings out a lot of passion from each side. There are also political matters and bills that have been passed that have made solving this issue harder. So, let's take look at the three psychologies of guns that make this issue so controversial.

Psychology I

A sector of our population fear guns, see zero need for them, and believe we would be far better off if civilians didn't own them...period. As with most views, it holds a certain amount of truth—no guns, no murders or suicides by guns. With the will to enact very strict laws, even criminals would be hard-pressed to get them; Japan, Australia and Britain are prime examples where death-rates by guns are in the low double-digits per year, in glaring contrast to America, a horrific 38,000 per year.

The people in this group fear the terrible finality guns pose, the ease at which they make possible to snuff out a life—a 1/4″ pull spells death—and that no so called "right to own" trumps the precious value of life. They feel there's no purpose to these instruments except to kill, with zero reconciliation for their existence in civilian life or to humanity. Their position is not altogether unfounded—a study in 2011 at the UCLA School of Public Health; among 23 high-income developed countries, 80% of all gun deaths, 86% of all women, and 87% of all children occurred in the U.S.

The proponents of very strict gun laws are frustrated because of their inability to understand why good decent people would want to have access to instruments of death, and they may believe that access to 911 is the only protection they need against a violent intruder, ignoring the fact that time is of the essence.

They see that gun violence is out of control and do not equate freedom with gun ownership, and would feel safer and freer without them.

Psychology II

The people in this group are mostly gun owners who of course believe in the Second Amendment for the right to own one, are responsible gun owners, and also support reasonable gun regulation like a viable comprehensive data base, a ban on semi-automatic military weapons because they feel these weapons make the country more dangerous (the Pew Center), a ban on large clips, and strict laws to dismantle the loophole where 40% of guns are acquired illegally.

The NRA certainly doesn't represent them, and they don't buy for a New York second the appalling hypocrisy of the NRA when it states, "Guns don't kill people, people kill people," then block any and every attempt to keep guns out of the hands of the wrong people. They are sickened by the massive gun-deaths our nation suffers each year, and it resonates with them when they hear a President ask, "Are we really prepared to say that we are powerless in the face of such carnage."

Their reason for gun ownership is to enjoy target shooting, hunting and home protection. They are equally balanced in both the rights to protect gun ownership and the importance of controlling gun ownership. The interesting fact about gun ownership is that the rate is double in the countryside than it is in the city, yet gun violence is for the most part, a city problem. This second group represents the overwhelming majority of gun owners.

Psychology III

The people here are also responsible gun owners and believe the prime purpose of owning guns is protection against government tyranny. Distrusting and suspecting their own government would betray the people. What is behind this suspicion and fear of people who continually envision this scenario, and further believe the only savior to this evil is to be well, even heavily armed? These are people who have lived in this wealthiest and most secure country in the world for decades, enjoying all the wonderful benefits it bestows upon them without any interruption of them in any form, yet they have formed a deep-seated paranoia of their government, believing it is poised to subjugate them at the first opportunity, to disarm them with the mental image of armed forces appearing at their door to confiscate their precious weapons—they being the only things that will save them from this perceived governmental enslavement. Their guns being the symbol of freedom, an undying, cherished notion that freedom is manifest in a bullet, clinging to their revered guns much as a child does a teddy bear.

They view the Second Amendment as the Holy Grail of the Constitution. While it is true the amendment was originally written with the intent to protect against the danger of a tyrannical government and probably was considered our first civic duty, it must be noted it was written at a time of monarchies, as our country was being subjugated by one. That is now an outdated and paranoid concern, as our government is based upon *We the People* for over two centuries.

This acute suspicion and anti-government phobia seems to be assuaged only by an abiding association with gun acquisition, inducing a sense of security as they envision themselves warding off any governmental assault with their weaponry. This premise is addressed directly in Sam Harris' article, *The Riddle of the Gun*, where he writes,

> [T]he idea that a few pistols and an AR 15 in every home constitutes a necessary bulwark against totalitarianism is fairly ridiculous. If you believe that the armed forces of the United States might one day come for you—and you think your cache of small arms will suffice to defend you if they do—I've got a black helicopter to sell you.

People of this group seem to be more susceptible to fear than most, having a defensive ideology, highly attuned to danger, with their antennae up for anything in their environment that seems threatening. By nature, we all have this sense to some degree, it comes from a little gland called the amygdala, and it's what kept our distant ancestors alive by alerting them to, and responding to danger by automatic response. Because it evolved over a time when danger was rampant everywhere, we have developed a "negativity bias." alive and well within us today.

Evolution favored those who were able to react with lightening speed, the amygdala taking over in order to save their lives, where in a situation of threat, it shuts down the ability to process information rationally as the nervous system reverts to automatic pilot for instantaneous protection. We have inherited that instinct; seemingly written into our DNA. As Dr. Rick Hanson, neuropsychologist and author puts it,

> The brain is like Velcro for everything negative and Teflon for the positives.

Some of us may have overly active or larger amygdalas heightening our sense of threat, and is inappropriate and counterproductive to existence in the modern world.

Tai Chi:
Highly Effective
Method of Improving
Balance and Equilibrium

The slow, deliberate footwork of the ancient Chinese martial art of tai chi has been shown to substantially improve balance, especially in older people, reducing their chance of falling. The movements bring a heightened awareness of the soles of the feet, changes in the angle of the ankle, and weight distribution. It also increases leg strength, flexibility, range of motion and reflexes. In the process of shifting your weight back and forth, the practitioner becomes increasingly adept at balancing in multiple positions, developing the ability to easily walk on uneven pavement or navigate busy walkways and shopping malls.

Tai chi is much more dynamic than it looks. Dr. Peter Wayne, is research director of the Osher Center for Integrative Medicine at Brigham and Women's Hospital and Harvard Medical School. He is also the founder and director of the Tree of Life Tai Chi Center in Somerville, Massachusetts. He states,

> The slowness that you see from the outside can be deceptive. Studies have shown tai chi to reduce falls in seniors by up to 45%.

Tai chi also makes you more aware of both your internal body and the external world, allowing you a far better sense of your position in space and therefore become much more stable. To boot, it is incredibly safe to practice.

New England Journal of Medicine Study

The New England Journal of Medicine conducted a study, *Tai Chi and Postural Stability in Patients with Parkinson's Disease*. The study compared three forms of exercise, tai chi, strength training and stretching to determine which of them best addressed balance. They assigned 195 patients from four Oregon cities into three of the different exercise groups. The patients participated in 60 minutes of exercise twice a week for 24 weeks. The protocol for tai chi consisted of six movements. The resistance training group focused on strengthening the muscles used for posture and balance, using weighted vests and ankle weights, involving 8 to 10 exercises. The stretching group did seated and standing stretches involving both the upper and lower body. The results were that,

> The participants in the tai chi group performed significantly better than those in the resistance-

training and stretching groups on the primary outcomes. The tai chi group had better performance than the resistance-training group. The tai chi group also had significantly better performance than the stretching group.

It is surprising, and counter intuitive, that an activity that looks and seems so gentle, relaxed and effortless in its execution can be so effective as to exceed the results of all the other exercise methods.

The History of Tai Chi

Tai chi is a martial art that is thousands of years old. The first known written reference of it appeared in the *Book of Changes* over 3000 years ago during the Zhou Dynasty (1100-1221 BC). The essential principles of Tai Chi are based on the ancient Chinese philosophy of Taoism, which stresses the natural balance in all things and the need for living in spiritual and physical harmony with the patterns of nature.

The philosophy of tai chi is based everything being composed of two opposites, and complementary elements of yin and yang, working in a relational harmony of perpetual balance. Tai chi consists of exercises equally balanced between yin and yang, in which the philosophy says makes it so remarkably effective.

In traditional Chinese medicine, human beings are considered miniature versions of the universe, and like the universe, they are thought to consist of an interaction of five elements—metal, water, fire, wood and earth, which integrate and flow through all the organs of the body, and is called qi (pronounced "chee"), or life force. This force, or energy, travels along pathways in the body called meridians. A state of good health is achieved when the interactions between these elements cause the flow of your qi to occur in a smooth, balanced and harmonious manner. The practice of tai chi is believed to help your qi flow smoothly.

How to Start

Dr. Peter Wayne authored a book that's available and inexpensive titled, *The Harvard Medical School Guide to Tai Chi: 12 Weeks to a Healthy Body, Strong Heart, and Sharp Mind,* for sale on many on line book stores. Also, there are many videos for beginners on youtube.com that you can select from, so take a look and have some fun viewing them to familiarize yourself with a few of the movements. This a great resource for you to learn, and with a little concentration and practice, you can put together a simple routine for yourself. If you can get YouTube on your TV, it would help greatly, where you can watch and practice along with the instructor. I myself learned from a video. One of the best beginner videos I've seen is *Tai Chi for Beginners* by Don Fiore. Web address is **https://www.youtube.com/watch?v=6L43 P1MY2KA&app=desktop**. It's an eight minute routine that is very easy to follow and do. Another way to learn tai chi would be to join a class offered in your community, where you would have a personal trainer guiding you.

Keep in mind, as a side benefit, you will be enhancing your brain function by learning a new activity as discussed in the chapter, *Grow Your*

Brain—Literally, on page 29. And remember that as in any endeavor consistency is where the magic is. Practicing tai chi right in your own home is very conducive to being consistent, deriving all the benefits attendant with it.